RE/INVENTION

Qualitative Methods "How-To" Guides
Patricia Leavy, Series Editor

This series offers researchers and students practical instruction on specific qualitative methods—what they are good for and how to use them in a study. All phases of research design are addressed: formulating a research question, hypothesis, and/or research purpose; developing a literature review; sampling; and collecting, analyzing, interpreting, and representing data. Evaluation criteria are considered and each method's historical and philosophical background is briefly described. With accessible writing and ample pedagogical features, books in the series are ideal for use in courses or by individual researchers.

Re/Invention: Methods of Social Fiction
Patricia Leavy

Re/Invention

METHODS OF SOCIAL FICTION

Patricia Leavy

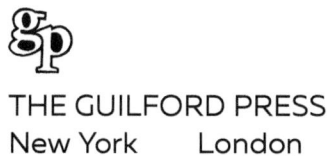

THE GUILFORD PRESS
New York   London

Copyright © 2023 The Guilford Press
A Division of Guilford Publications, Inc.
370 Seventh Avenue, Suite 1200, New York, NY 10001
www.guilford.com

All rights reserved

No part of this book may be reproduced, translated, stored in a retrieval system, or transmitted, in any form or by any means, electronic, mechanical, photocopying, microfilming, recording, or otherwise, without written permission from the publisher.

Printed in the United States of America

This book is printed on acid-free paper.

Last digit is print number: 9 8 7 6 5 4 3 2 1

Library of Congress Cataloging-in-Publication Data is available from the publisher.

ISBN 978-1-4625-4768-5 (paperback) — ISBN 978-1-4625-5029-6 (hardcover)

For the trailblazing scholars who inspire me, with gratitude:

Yichien Cooper, Carolyn Ellis, Rita Irwin, and Laurel Richardson

Preface

I've loved creative writing since I was a little girl. When I was about 10 years old, I had a wonderful English teacher, Miss Mercer. She encouraged my writing. With her support, I actually tried to write a novel—an epic love story about people who help each other heal. Because I was 10, it didn't pan out. However, my passion for writing never lessened, and decades later that book would be written. There was much I loved about creating fictional worlds—finding refuge, escape, and solace; feeling less lonely; meeting new people, caring for them, and learning about their lives; making connections that had previously been invisible; figuring things out I wouldn't otherwise understand; acknowledging the unfair and painful dimensions of life; imagining how things might be different; and more.

From the time I was very young, I wanted to be a writer, a novelist. The truth is I was too afraid to pursue my passion. Making a career in the arts is tough. There's so much rejection and critique. It takes courage and vulnerability, both of which I lacked. Fearing I couldn't handle it, I chose another path, earned a doctorate degree in sociology, and became a professor. As a result, I started publishing nonfiction academic work. I look back now and laugh because my first journal articles, published when I was in graduate school, were deeply grounded in the arts and creative writing. There was nothing traditional about them. They were artistic and experimental. Somehow, as I continued down the academic path, my writing became less creative and increasingly conventional. My work also started to feel like *work*. Soon after I realized that if I didn't enjoy what I was writing, why would anyone enjoy reading it? People often talk about going down a dark spiral, but this realization did the opposite for me; it sent me down a spiral of lightness. I began to look seriously at the nature of academic research and reporting. Does anyone read this stuff? Is it any good? Does it affect people outside of the academy? Yes, my spiral was one of awareness. It was a reality check, a gut check. Life is too short to waste our time and other resources conducting research that does little more than serve as a line on our CV. Through this process of reflection on the nature of academic publishing and my own work, I found my courage and turned to the arts. For me this wasn't so much a turn, but a re/turn. After spending several years immersed in arts-based research, I wrote my first novel and soon thereafter quit my tenured teaching gig. More than a dozen novels later, I've never looked back.

Arts-Based Research

Arts-based research (ABR) draws on the creative arts as a legitimate way of knowing. ABR involves researchers in any discipline adapting the tenets of the creative arts in their research projects in order to address research problems in holistic ways. The arts practice may be used during any phase of the research—data generation, analysis, interpretation, and representation—or it may be used as the entire method of inquiry. Arts-based practices may draw on any art form: literary, performative, or visual. ABR opens up new ways of thinking and seeing, allows us to ask and answer new questions or address old questions in new ways, and can illuminate that which would otherwise remain in darkness. While researchers have long been using fiction as a way of knowing, as reviewed in Chapter 2, the method of "social fiction," a term I coined in 2010, developed within the context of the emergent ABR paradigm.

Why This Book Is Needed

I wrote this book as an in-depth introduction to social fiction. During the dozen years I've been publishing novels and other works of fiction, I've also been documenting this methodology in the hopes of providing a road map for others, one that I've largely had to figure out on my own. Even though many scholars have long been writing fiction, others have not provided methods texts for those still wishing to learn this approach to inquiry. In addition to my own writing, I also created and served as editor for the *Social Fictions* book series, the first and only book series published by an academic press that produces full-length literary works written by scholars. During my decade-long tenure as editor, over 40 books were published and I reviewed countless submissions. This was also a tremendous learning experience and one that showed me that the field has grown enormously. There's other evidence of the rise in social fiction as well, including numerous sessions at national and international conferences across the disciplines, the development of SoFi, an online zine created by sociologist Ash Watson, and increased journal publications (recently *Art/Research International: A Transdisciplinary Journal [ARI]* had a special issue on "Fiction as Research" guest edited by Ash Watson and Jessica Smartt Gullion). Personal encounters have also fueled my desire to write this book. I've had many experiences on the road after delivering keynotes, lectures, and workshops at universities about social fiction. Likewise, I regularly join classes virtually to talk about my novels and fiction as a research practice. Based on all these interactions, it has become clear to me that a contemporary book on this method is needed. Those informal conversations have guided my thinking as I developed a structure for this book. I hope to show you that social fiction is a valid and exciting method of inquiry and to encourage you to develop your own practice, so that you can create the story-worlds and characters that inhabit them that could not come from anyone else.

Organization of This Book

This book includes in-depth introductory chapters as well as excerpts from my published works of social fiction accompanied by original reflections on those excerpts. The pairing of the introductory review chapters with published social fiction provides a context for understanding fiction as a research practice as well as examples of its use. Chapters 1–3 provide background on writing as inquiry, the historical and contemporary context for social fiction, and detailed instruction on how to write social fiction. Chapters 4–8 are divided into the different structures fiction writers use. The structures covered are traditional three-act structures, sequels, series, open form structures, alternative structures, and short stories. Each of these chapters includes an introduction explaining the literary structure, a reprinted extract from one of my works of fiction (the set-up is provided), and a reflection on each extract that highlights techniques reviewed in Chapter 3, so you can see them in action. I was inspired to include examples of my own work with original reflections after reading *Revision: Autoethnographic Reflections on Life and Work* by Carolyn Ellis, in which she uses a similar format. Using my own work, as Ellis did, allowed me to include personal details about the source of my inspiration, the writing process, and my intent. Finally, Chapter 9 offers practical advice on publishing fiction as well as evaluation criteria.

In addition to including in-depth introductory chapters, examples of published social fiction, and reflections on the writing process, each chapter in this book includes "tip bubbles" with additional hints for those wanting to write social fiction. There are also two types of exercises at the end of every chapter. Skill-building exercises are meant for students learning about this method and are intended to help you begin to develop a writing practice using the strategies and techniques in this book. Rethink-your-research exercises are meant for researchers already engaged in research. They are intended to help you reimagine your research as fiction—whether you decide to use the method for your current project or to develop ideas and skills for future projects. There is also an appendix with suggested readings.

Alternative Ways of Reading This Book

Although this book can be read in order from beginning to end, it need not be. Each introductory chapter can be read on its own; so too can the reprinted works of fiction. Therefore, readers interested in particular fictional formats can read just those pertinent chapters. It's also important to note that many of the extracted works of fiction serve dual purposes. For example, the excerpts from my novels *Blue* and *Film* are reprinted in Chapter 5, which focuses on sequels. However, they are also examples of using a traditional three-act structure. Furthermore, they include examples of techniques, such as interiority, dialogue, and flashbacks. So even if you have no interest in writing a sequel, the exemplars may still be of use. Likewise, the excerpts from the Tess Lee and Jack Miller novels reprinted in Chapter 6 are both examples of writing a series and using an open form structure. Even if you don't intend to write a series, most fiction writers find it useful to learn how to write in open form.

Audience for This Book

This book is accessibly written for diverse audiences, including undergraduates, graduates, researchers, scholars, writers, and practitioners interested in social fiction. In terms of teaching, this book can be used in courses in communications, creative arts therapy, creative writing, cultural studies, education, expressive therapies, health studies, social work, sociology, psychology, theatre arts, and women's, gender, and sexuality studies. It can be used in methodology courses, such as ABR, qualitative research, survey of research methods, emergent research practices, narrative inquiry, and critical approaches to research.

Rest assured, this book is not intended only for those who already have training in writing fiction. I appreciate that sometimes, for all sorts of reasons, it can be scary to work with new approaches, especially in artistic forms that require a certain level of vulnerability and bravery. I encourage you to go ahead and try anyway. Begin from where you are. Candidly, when I wrote my first novel, *Low-Fat Love*, I knew nothing about what I was doing. What I had was a desire to try to do it—to get my insights and the stories of those I interviewed out in a new, more engaging, and accessible way. The rewards have been well beyond anything I could have imagined. My work and life have never been the same. I had a new path forward. I hope this book provides the same for you.

ACKNOWLEDGMENTS

First and foremost, heartfelt thanks to my extraordinary editor and dear friend C. Deborah Laughton. You are a gift! Your wisdom is reflected on every page. Any errors are all my own. A spirited thank-you to Seymour Weingarten, Bob Matloff, Judith Grauman, Anna Brackett, Katherine Lieber, Marian Robinson, Paul Gordon, Andrea Sargent, and the entire Guilford Press team. I am grateful for the feedback of the following reviewers: Barbara Dennis, School of Education, Indiana University; Jessica Smartt Gullion, College of Arts and Sciences, Texas Woman's University; Candace Stout, Department of Arts Administration, Education, and Policy, The Ohio State University; Kenya E. Wolff, Department of Early Childhood Education, University of Mississippi; and Sandra Faulkner, School of Media and Communication, Bowling Green State University. Shalen Lowell, you are the world's best assistant. I also extend deep appreciation to Clear Voice Editors for their incredible copyediting work on many of the fictional works excerpted in this book. Likewise, thank you to the original publishing teams for the excerpted works. I am grateful to you all. I couldn't do this work without a good support system. My deep gratitude to my friends and colleagues, especially Tony Adams, Vanessa Alssid, Melissa Anyiwo, Keith Berry, Celine Boyle, Renita Davis, Pamela DeSantis, Ally Field, Alexandra Lasczik, Xan Nowakowski, Laurel Richardson, Mr. Barry Shuman, Eve Spangler, and J. E. Sumerau. Thanks as always to my family. Mark, I appreciate your support more than I can say. Madeline, you are my heart and a beautiful writer in your own right. Finally I dedicate this book to four trailblazing scholars—artists and writers—who continue to pave the way for so many others with their courageous and innovative work: Yichien Cooper, Carolyn Ellis, Rita Irwin, and Laurel Richardson. You inspire me beyond measure. Thank you for your generosity.

PERMISSIONS

The following works of fiction are reprinted in this book with permission:

Leavy, P. (2016). *Blue*. Rotterdam, The Netherlands: Sense Publishers. Copyright © 2016 Patricia Leavy. Reprinted with permission of the author.

Leavy, P., & Scotti, V. (2017). *Low-Fat Love Stories*. Rotterdam, The Netherlands: Sense Publishers. Copyright © 2017 Patricia Leavy. Reprinted with permission of the author.

Leavy, P. (2019). *Spark*. New York: Guilford Press. Copyright © 2019 The Guilford Press. Reprinted with permission of The Guilford Press.

Leavy, P. (2020). *Film*. Leiden, The Netherlands: Brill. Copyright © 2020 Patricia Leavy. Reprinted with permission of the author.

Leavy, P. (2020). *Shooting Stars*. Leiden, The Netherlands: Brill. Copyright © 2020 Patricia Leavy. Adapted with permission of the author.

Leavy, P. (2021). *Twinkle*. Leiden, The Netherlands: Brill. Copyright © 2021 Patricia Leavy. Reprinted with permission of the author.

Leavy, P. (2021). *Constellations*. Leiden, The Netherlands: Brill. Copyright © 2021 Patricia Leavy. Reprinted with permission of the author.

Leavy, P. (2021). *Low-Fat Love: 10th Anniversary Edition*. Kennebunk, ME: Paper Stars Press. Copyright © 2021 Patricia Leavy. Reprinted with permission of the author.

Leavy, P. (2021). *Supernova*. Leiden, The Netherlands: Brill. Copyright © 2021 Patricia Leavy. Reprinted with permission of the author.

Leavy, P. (2022). *North Star*. Kennebunk, ME: Paper Stars Press. Copyright © 2022 Patricia Leavy. Reprinted with permission of the author.

Contents

1 Writing as Inquiry   1
  Social Fiction *3*
  The Creative Writing Process and Being a Creative *4*
  The Strengths of Social Fiction *8*
  Conclusion *16*

2 Historical and Contemporary Context for Social Fiction   18
  Fiction in the Humanities and Social Sciences *19*
  Historical Fiction *22*
  Creative Nonfiction *26*
  Qualitative Research *28*
  Arts-Based Research *32*
  Literary Neuroscience *34*
  Public Scholarship *36*
  Challenges of Doing Fiction as Research *38*
  Conclusion *40*
  Notes *40*

3 The Method: How to Write Social Fiction   42
  Generating Ideas, Themes, and Data *43*
  Building a Structure *46*
  Style *52*
  Characterization *55*
  Literary Tools *59*
  Front and Back Matter *64*
  Titles *65*
  Conclusion *66*

4 Traditional Three-Act Structures   68

Low-Fat Love   69
Low-Fat Love, Excerpt from Chapter 4   71
Low-Fat Love, Excerpt from Chapter 7   78
Low-Fat Love, Excerpt from Chapter 18   81
Reflection on *Low-Fat Love*   83

5 Sequels: More on Traditional Three-Act Structures   87

Blue   88
Blue, Chapter 1   89
Reflection on *Blue*   96
Film   98
Film, Chapter 10   99
Reflection on *Film*   106
Notes   108

6 Series and Open Form Structures   109

Celestial Bodies: The Tess Lee and Jack Miller Novels   111
Shooting Stars   112
Shooting Stars, Chapter 1   113
Reflection on *Shooting Stars*   121
Twinkle   123
Twinkle, Chapter 4   123
Reflection on *Twinkle*   147
Constellations   149
Constellations Epilogue, "The Next Day"   150
Reflection on *Constellations*   154
Supernova   154
Supernova, Excerpt from Chapter 8   155
Reflection on *Supernova*   156
North Star   156
North Star, Chapter 4   157
Reflection on *North Star*   161
Reflection on *Celestial Bodies: The Tess Lee and Jack Miller Novels*   162

7 Alternative Structures   167

Spark   169
Spark, Excerpt from Chapter 8   171
Reflection on *Spark*   178

8 Short Stories   181

Low-Fat Love Stories   182
Low-Fat Love Stories, Chapter 10, "Mirror Mirror"   185
Reflection on Low-Fat Love Stories   189
Notes   190

9 Practical Advice for Publishing and Evaluating Social Fiction   191

Publishing Fiction   192
Awards   196
Evaluation Criteria   197
Conclusion   205

Appendix: Recommended Reading   207

Education   207
Gender   207
LGBTQIA   207
Race/Multiculturalism   207
Pandemics/Quarantine   208

References   209

Index   215

About the Author   224

1 Writing as Inquiry

> *Literature reveals that we are the possibilities of ourselves.*
> —WOLFGANG ISER

Much of my childhood was spent in story-worlds. I loved reading, listening to stories, and, above all, writing. There was magic to be found in fictional worlds—they transported me to different places even when I was sitting in my bedroom. I'd meet new people, learn about their lives, feel their pain and joy, and carry their lessons with me, as if they were now a part of my blueprint and my world. Creative writing was a refuge that allowed me to express ideas that were otherwise just out of reach. By writing fiction, I could take my experiences and observations, mix them up in a mental blender with imagination and fantasy, and suddenly have something that didn't exist before. The possibilities to explore and document life as I knew it and life as I could imagine it were infinite.

Despite my passion for fiction, I chose another path professionally, and became an academic. As a sociologist I was still engaged in exploring human experience and trying to make sense of the world, and I was still writing, although the format was prescribed, formulaic, and limited. Like many in the academy, I was taught that writing is something we do *as we do something else*—something bigger, our actual work. Out of sheer frustration, I began to question this system, and to write on the borders of it. Eventually I realized that writing didn't need to be an addendum to my scholarly pursuit, that it's a part of all research and can even constitute research.

Researchers from all paradigms engage in writing from the outset of any project—jotting down ideas, taking notes on literature, drafting proposals, sending emails, constructing invitations to participants and collaborators, and so on. Writing continues through data generation, analysis, interpretation, and the representation of research findings. It's intertwined with the entire research process. In academia, writing is generally understood to *facilitate* inquiry. It's something we do as a part of the research process and a method for communicating research findings. However, writing can be so much more.

Qualitative researcher Harry F. Wolcott astutely noted that writing doesn't merely reflect thinking, but rather "writing is thinking" (2009, p. 8). Similarly, sociologist Laurel Richardson (2000) has explained that writing helps us discover what we think. Therefore, writing can be understood as a process of discovery in its own right. That is the starting point for this book. I'm particularly interested in how writing fiction can be a research practice in its own right—simultaneously a method of inquiry and of representation.

Fiction draws us in to new yet familiar worlds in which we might meet strangers or characters that serve as reflections of pieces of ourselves. Through the pleasure found in immersing ourselves in resonant story-worlds, the process of reading fiction can be transformative, as is the process of writing it. Fiction is engaged.

Fiction is both a form of writing and a way of reading (Cohn, 2000). We write fiction differently from how we write nonfiction—with literary tools, attention to aesthetics, and the freedom that comes from imagination. We read it differently too—with our defenses down, with our emotions at the forefront, with a suspension of disbelief, and with the assumption that as a leisure time activity we are just as qualified to read it as anyone else. It's for everyone. Fiction grants us an imaginary entry into what is otherwise inaccessible. The practices of writing and reading fiction allow us to access imaginary or possible worlds, to reexamine the worlds we live in, and to enter into the psychological processes that motivate people and the sociohistorical realities that shape them. Central to understanding the power of fiction, we must bear two things in mind. First, fiction allows writers to both chronicle or document experience *and* to reimagine it. Through fiction we can revisit the past, explore the present, and imagine the future. Second, readers come to care about characters as if they're people—they become invested in them. We journey with them. For these reasons, which are elaborated throughout this book, engaging with fiction in our research practice creates innumerable possibilities.

Social Fiction

As reviewed in the next chapter, combining fiction and academic research concerns is not new. There's a rich history of scholars using literary writing as a means of developing and communicating their theories and ideas. Consider, for example, Jean-Paul Sartre, Simone de Beauvoir, Zora Neale Hurston, whose work is discussed in the following chapter. They each wrote many novels, novellas, short stories, plays, and other creative works espousing their research. Sartre was even awarded the Nobel Prize in Literature for this very kind of work. There are countless other examples, including many who are lesser known. The contemporary move toward fiction as a research practice thus is not a turn, but a re/turn. It's interesting because, as might be expected, there is pushback to the idea of fiction as a research practice, as if it's a shocking, new, and "out there" innovation. Yet history shows otherwise. It's always been there, and in select cases, highly regarded. This is a lesson we need to learn over and over again. The literary arts can be powerful for scholars. Perhaps part of the reason we need to relearn this simple lesson is that the works of literature created by scholars always appear as individual cases that aren't linked in any way. They occur at different times and in different fields—historical fiction, philosophical fiction, science fiction (written by STEM scholars), dystopian fiction (written by social scientists), and so on. My aim is to find a way to name and house all this work.

How can we describe the work scholars do when they use literary writing to convey intellectual concerns or research findings? In 2010, after penning my debut novel, I coined the term "social fiction." By social fiction I mean fiction that is written by researchers in any field and reflects their social research concerns or expertise. A work of social fiction may be based on a particular study in the traditional sense, or it may be influenced by the author's cumulative insights and perspective.

How can we distinguish social fiction from generic fiction? This is a question I'm often asked. It's about *intent* and *perspective*. What is your intent in writing the piece? What perspective or lens do you bring to bear? Rebecca Hussey (2021) suggests that philosophical fiction "deals with ideas in a direct way." She goes on to explain that while this description could apply to any work of fiction, it's about "degree." She explains that philosophical fiction purposely provokes readers to contemplate big questions. Similarly, sociologist Ash Watson suggests that sociological fictions "intentionally engage with sociological foci and ways of thinking"

(2021, p. 5). She further explains that sociological fiction explores sociological understandings and is grounded in sociological knowledge (Watson, 2021, p. 6). The same is true for social fiction. What I like about the term social fiction is that it's not bound to any one discipline and thus can be used to describe all the diverse work scholars do as they create fiction, both past and present. I'm always quick to point out that despite naming the practice, I did not invent social fiction. It's not a new invention. It's a re/invention.

The Creative Writing Process and Being a Creative

People often ask me if I consider myself first a scholar or a novelist. I am both at once. I've come to believe that all intellectuals and artists share something in common—at the core, we are creatives. Part of understanding how art can be research centers on considering the architecture of knowledge. What shapes might knowledge take (Leavy, 2011)? Literary writing is one such shape. For me, social fiction is my way of understanding the topics I explore, developing and shaping my insights, and sharing them. Writing is my conceptual frame. It is my inquiry, my investigation, and my final synthesis, the representation of the creative process. Many social fiction authors explain their inquiry similarly. Using an art form as an entire research act is not limited to the literary arts either. For example, Barbara J. Fish is a visual artist. She makes response art as an act of research and analysis, and it serves to represent the entire process. Fish writes: "The process of drawing, painting, and investigating the response art that I create about what I witness is my research. The images are the vehicle of investigation, as well as its synthesis" (2018, p. 339).

We all approach a literary arts practice differently, so I'll briefly share how I came to mine. Despite my lifelong love of creative writing and the dabbling or experimenting I did throughout graduate school and my early career, it was not until writing my first novel that I fully embraced writing fiction as a research practice. My reasons for writing the novel are hardly poetic; they were pragmatic. I was frustrated and needed a better way to communicate with audiences.

For nearly a decade I collected interview research, primarily with women, about their relationships, gender and sexual identities, body image, self-esteem, and related topics. I wrote peer-reviewed articles and presented my work at professional conferences. It was impossible to shake the persistent feeling that these formats didn't capture the essence of what I had learned over the years, nor were they accessible to anyone outside of the academy. These women's stories were emotional, textured, layered, and relatable. None of that was coming through. Moreover, I had my own life experiences that informed my thinking, with no place to share those insights. Honestly, I was bored and uninspired. If I felt that way as the author, what could I expect from anyone else? My frustration led me to arts-based research (ABR) and ultimately social fiction.

Drawing on insights gleaned from my research participants as well as personal experiences and observations, I decided to take everything I had learned that didn't seem to have a home and put it into a fictional work. This was the inspiration for my debut novel *Low-Fat Love* (discussed in-depth in Chapter 4). Through the fictional format I was able to deliver the content, layer themes, sensitively portray composite characters, create empathetic understandings, promote self-reflection in readers, create longer-lasting learning experiences for readers, and most important, get the work out to academic *and* lay audiences. For more than a decade, I have spoken about the novel to students at universities, virtually joined book clubs for Q&As with readers from all walks of life, and received emails from readers. What I have been most struck by is how deeply readers have been affected by the novel.

My initial turn to a literary arts practice stemmed from sociological concerns. However, over the years inspiration has come in many different forms, the seeds for projects developing in new ways. When asked how I come up with ideas for my novels, my answer is always the same: it never happens the same way twice, which is why I'm still in love with writing. Sometimes I get a complete idea. I'll have some experience, make ethnographic observations, or even just hear a song or see a painting and an entire story comes to me, from beginning to end, complete with characters, and it unfolds in my mind like a movie. My job is to transcribe it. At other times I just get a little spark of an idea. For example, a character will come to me, and that's the starting point. Sometimes there's a topic or theme I want to explore. I may conduct research and/or read literature, and then I'll try to build a character and plot around the central themes. Or there will be a structure I want to use. For example, one of my novels came about because I wanted to build a before–together–after story structure that allowed me to explore the effect of group happenings on individuals (elaborated in Chapter 7). In this structure, characters are first shown in their own lives, then they are all together and something happens, and then they are again shown in their own lives affected by their time together. I stewed on the idea, trying to come up with a story that served that structure. Then I watched a movie and a song came on. Suddenly I knew the characters and the plot. This isn't unusual for me. Often my exposure to a piece of art will serve as the inspiration for a novel. I'll hear a song, see a painting, or watch a film, and a new story emerges. Like I said, it never happens the same way twice, which makes it magical.

If you're not sure how you would even find a general topic to explore, here are some strategies to try:

- Make a list of topics you're interested in, based on what you're learning in school and/or personal interests and experiences.
- Make a list of social justice issues you care about.
- Make a list of current events you think are important.

In Chapter 3 I offer additional advice for how to start a social fiction project so you're not just sitting around waiting for inspiration to strike—sometimes it happens that way, but not always. For now, I'd like to further explore the role of magic in creative writing and also how art can inspire art.

Virginia Woolf had a point when she said that we need time and our own space in order to write, but there are ways to make do with scraps of time and, for that matter, scraps of paper. So what does it take for any of us to write fiction? Discipline? Training? Skill? Divine inspiration? Magic? Maybe a little of each. To me, it all comes down to a balance of discipline and magic. Some novelists say that all writing is discipline, because they want to remind people it's hard work and they want to encourage novices that they can do it. Other novelists say it's all magic and "visits from the muses," because they want people to believe they are uniquely talented. The truth is, it's both. Moreover, discipline prepares us for magic. Allow me to explain.

Creative writing demands discipline. It's a rigorous craft that must be learned and practiced. Many days will be spent plodding away, forcing yourself to do the work, even when it isn't particularly fun. But there's magic too. It can't be planned. This is because writing is a process of discovery and creation. How does magic happen? Discipline brings it on and allows us to take full advantage of it when the moment presents itself. By learning the tools of our craft, honing our writing skills through rigorous practice, and even forcing ourselves to write when it's hard, understanding we can edit later when the magical bits happen, we're ready. Sometimes writing fiction really is hard work, and we just go word by word, line by line. At other times we're so swept up, we may forget to eat lunch. There's a creative elixir fueling us. That's the best part. When magic strikes, whether we're watching a movie or listening to a song and characters start to appear before us, or we're already deep into a project and suddenly a character says something unexpected and we go with it, that's the divine part. Both the discipline and the magic it will bring are available to us all—to you just as they are to me. Work hard and be ready.

To be a creative, we must engage with creativity, not just our own. Many writers look to the arts in seeking inspiration. I've already shared how a song in a film planted the seeds for one of my novels. It's important for writers to actively use the arts. Listen to music, look at visual art, watch films, television, or live performances. But don't expect that because you look at a painting suddenly a short story will unfurl itself before you. That can happen, but usually it's not linear. The ideas you develop as you experience art may influence your writing in all kinds of ways. Expose yourself to art and artists. One thing I've done for nearly every novel I've written is to create a musical playlist. Sometimes the songs actually find their way onto the pages, but more often they simply provide a soundscape for me—they help put me in the mood of the story-world. Many novelists use music in similar ways. Sometimes art in a different medium can even help you understand your own medium better. For example, when I was working on a collection of short stories based on qualitative interview research with women (discussed in Chapter 8), I intentionally listened to songs by female singer-songwriters, including in genres I don't normally enjoy, like country music. The kinds of songs those musicians create aligned with my goals of creating very brief stories with layers of meaning. Again inspiration can come to us in many ways, but sometimes it's best not to sit around waiting for it and to actively seek it out.

> If you're working on a piece of fiction and looking for inspiration or a new way to think about it, seek out examples in other art forms. For instance, if you're trying to write a character profile, view paintings of portraits, read monologues from plays, or listen to songs by confessional singers. Inspiration is not linear in the sense that A will cause B, but you may unlock some new pathways of thinking and seeing. Inspiration is complex. Seek it out. Lean into it.

Being a creative requires discipline, flexibility, and thinking in new ways. It requires us to look at our arts practice as a process of discovery and to remain open to the unknown, the magical bits we could never plan. It also requires us to delve deep into our imaginations, hunt for words and their meanings, and trust the insights we unearth. There's no getting around the fact that putting our fiction into the world also makes us vulnerable. Writers must be brave—both in their writing and in their willingness to share it come what may (this point is elaborated in later chapters). How we each approach the creative writing process, how we each embody the identity of a creative, and how we navigate sharing our work is entirely personal. I share my experiences and what I've learned only to provide some examples, but the possibilities are limitless.

Why do all this? Why turn to the literary arts in your research? As you'll see, there are many benefits to writing social fiction.

The Strengths of Social Fiction

Overall social fiction allows us to sensitively portray human experience in a way that often is difficult or impossible with traditional research practices in which participants are reduced to numbers or carefully curated excerpts from transcripts. Human experience is multidimensional, nuanced, complex, and situated in sociohistorical contexts and constellations of interpersonal relationships. It's messy. The way we live life is rarely the way researchers report on our lives, simply because of the tools and formats they're using. Storytelling, the basis of social fiction, can help address these issues. Narrative researchers understand this principle. Ruthellen Josselson (2006) has explained that narrative can be used to preserve the complexity of human experience, which may otherwise be lost or rendered invisible. Similarly Arthur P. Bochner and Andrew Herrmann (2020) suggest that narrative can be used to humanize our work. All the strengths of social fiction outlined in this chapter contribute to the larger goal of humanizing our understanding and the portrayal of human experience.

As I review the primary strengths of social fiction, please know that this list is by no means exhaustive. I want to note up-front that I do not discuss how fiction can aid public scholarship, and not because this issue is not relevant. On the contrary, I believe it is one of the most important functions that social fiction can serve. Traditional academic research is completely inaccessible to the public and even poorly read within the academy. Fiction can bridge the long divide between academia and the multiple publics in which we are enmeshed and that we wish to serve. The only reason I do not discuss public scholarship as a strength of social fiction is because it is obvious and well established. Traditional academic reporting belongs to the few; fiction is available to the many. Clearly that is a strength. In the next chapter, I do address how the push toward public scholarship has fostered the recent rise in social fiction. Finally I discuss verisimilitude at greater length because it is a necessary precondition for any of the other outcomes. We must create authentic story-worlds if we hope to reach readers in the other ways I've reviewed.

Verisimilitude

Verisimilitude refers to the creation of a realistic, authentic, resonant, and lifelike portrayal of people and settings. In other words, verisimilitude centers on truthfully portraying human experience. It rings true. Achieving verisimilitude is a standard goal in qualitative research and one of the benchmarks against which ethnographies, for instance, are evaluated. Fiction is uniquely suited for capturing verisimilitude.

In reading a work of fiction, if the author has achieved verisimilitude, we suspend our disbelief and become swept up in the story-world—its sights, sounds, and people. Whether the fictional worlds and the characters we are introduced to are similar or dissimilar to us, we are meant to step into their reality, become immersed in it, and accept the story-world. This is a marker of verisimilitude. The way someone's home is decorated, the smells coming out of their kitchen, the thoughts racing through their mind, and the conversations they have with their loved ones all contribute to a sense of reality or realness. I say "realness" because it's irrelevant whether the reality portrayed is Times Square in New York City in 2021 or on an imaginary planet in the future. It isn't about whether or not the story-world is a real place, it's about readers' acceptance of the story-world as a possible reality. It feels authentic, and we buy it. That's verisimilitude.

There is an immediacy to fiction that other forms of representation lack (Banks, 2008). Fiction writers go to great lengths, including conducting extensive research, to achieve realism and resonance (Banks, 2008; Berger, 1977). Wolfgang Iser writes: "In the novel, then the real and the possible coexist" (1997, p. 5). As researchers, we meticulously incorporate real-world details into the construction of fictional worlds. This allows us to both create realism and build "possible worlds" that may not exist as such (Banks & Banks, 1998). In this way we can present something that is authentic while also inviting readers to imagine the world differently. We can chronicle the way things are *and* we can imagine how things might be. As Iser suggests, the act of fictionalizing can make "conceivable what would otherwise remain hidden" (1997, p. 4).

H. Porter Abbott (2008) suggests that social reality and our perception of it are inextricably intertwined with our engagement with the worlds constructed in fiction. He writes:

> The question of how our understanding of the actual world we live in, including history, plays a part in the made-up worlds of fiction. And the answer to the question is that our understanding of this actual world plays a huge part in almost all fictional worlds. In fact, unless we are told otherwise, we assume that the fictional world is a simulacrum of the world we actually live in. (p. 151)

Marie-Laure Ryan coined the term "principle of minimal departure," which refers to the assumption that the world in fiction resonates with our own reality unless the text itself tells us otherwise (Abbott, 2008). S. Christian Wheeler, Melanie C. Green, and Timothy C. Brock note that authors may attempt to achieve verisimilitude through the use of "familiar elements such as local settings, famous personages, and commonly known events" (1999, p. 136). In other words, by using elements that are "real" or "familiar," writers create a sense of believability. Many social fiction authors believe their work has scholarly merit because they have created an authentic "possible reality." For example, Peter Clough (2002) presents five fictional stories occurring in educational settings. He suggests that the stories are legitimate pieces of research because they *could have happened*. Here we can see how the realistic, authentic, or plausible nature of the texts—their ability to correspond with "reality"—is central to the research practice.

Iser has been at the forefront of theorizing about the relationship between the empirical worlds we study and the fictional worlds we create. His concept of "overstepping" indicates that a "literary work oversteps the real world which it incorporates" (1997, p. 1). Iser has detailed a threefold fictionalizing process: (1) selection, (2) combination, and (3) self-disclosure.

Selection is the process of taking "identifiable items" from social reality, importing them into the fictional world, and transforming them "into a sign for something other than themselves" (Iser, 1997, p. 2).

Through the process of selection, we "overstep" the empirical world we aim to reference. Selection happens in conjunction with combination.

Combination is the process of bringing the different empirical elements or details together. The bits of data, empirical elements, or details we select may be derived from traditional research processes (such as interviews or field research), or they may emerge through the process of writing itself. Tom Barone and Elliot W. Eisner explained that empirical details may arise out of any social research methods, and they further suggested that "empirical elements may also arise out of careful reflections on the previous experiences of the researcher with social phenomena. The research may occur within a preproduction phase, prior to the fashioning of a text; more often it will occur within the process of composition" (2012, p. 104). Therefore the descriptions and details contained in social fiction can be considered data. The use of details from the real world brings readers into the work of fiction while allowing writers to reimagine what real worlds are. According to Barone and Eisner: "Familiar elements of experience do help to lure the reader into the text and enable her to vicariously inhabit the world recreated therein. . . . The imported 'realities' . . . must nevertheless remain identifiable and familiar, seen as believable, credible, lest readers no longer be able to relate the recreated world to their life experiences outside of the text" (2012, p. 106).

According to Iser (1997), the final act of fictionalizing is self-disclosure. Self-disclosure refers to the ways that a text reveals or conceals its fictional nature (Barone & Eisner, 2012). When a text discloses its fictional nature, as literary texts do through various conventions (which may be as simple as labeling the work a novel), readers engage with it accordingly. Iser has suggested that when readers consume fictional works they engage in a process of "bracketing" whereby the real world or empirical reality is bracketed off from the fictional world. In other words, readers create a boundary between what they perceive to be the real world they are enmeshed in and the fictional world they are being invited into. Through this process readers are able to take the fictional world as an "as if" world (Iser, 1997, p. 3). Iser summarizes the fictionalizing process as follows:

> The acts of fictionalizing can be clearly distinguished by the different gestalt each of them brings about: selection results in revealing the intentionality of the author; combination results in bringing about unfamiliar relationships of the items selected within the text; and self-disclosure results in bracketing the world represented, thereby converting it into

a sign for something else, and simultaneously suspending the reader's natural attitude (1997, p. 4)

While trying to capture verisimilitude, it is also necessary to keep the bigger picture in mind. Whereas the details included in the story are important, the larger narrative is what readers are left with, and it must ring true and connect with them. The details are there to assist with the larger narrative. In fiction, meaning extends beyond individual facts (Abbott, 2008). Aristotle thought that the kind of truth that can live in fiction is a philosophical, universal truth that is far more powerful than any other form of truth (Abbott, 2008, pp. 153–154). So, though details help us achieve verisimilitude, the overall meaning constructed in fictional stories is greater than the sum of its parts.

Empathetic Understanding

Perhaps more than anything else a compassionate research practice, which is the cornerstone of social justice research, requires the cultivation of empathy, or learning about and feeling for others, however similar or dissimilar they may be from us. Empathy means we understand and care for others. Daniel Goleman (1995) famously notes in his best-selling book that empathy is a critical component of "emotional intelligence." Reading fiction can foster empathy. Rishma Dunlop states that "we write ourselves as we read" (2001, p. 12).

Many researchers aim at promoting empathy as a means of creating understanding. Fiction is well suited to eliciting empathy and promoting "empathetic engagement" (de Freitas, 2003). As readers engage with fiction and develop highly personal relationships with the characters, they are in fact constructing intimate relationships with "the imagined other" (de Freitas, 2003, p. 5). It doesn't take academic research to tell us that readers come to care about fictional characters, sometimes deeply. Anyone who has ever read a novel already knows that. Why do we care about fictional characters? What is the nature of that caring, and how does it contribute to empathetic or sympathetic engagement?

Wayne Booth suggested that we care about fictional characters "as human beings" (1961, p. 130). We want things to go well for those characters we come to love (Booth, 1961). Eileen John (2016) looks at this subject a little differently, suggesting we care about characters as *representations*. We are emotionally invested, as if we have a stake in how things work out for them (Booth, 1961; John, 2016; Robinson, 2005). We may even root for characters that are not sympathetic in some ways (Robinson, 2005). What's most interesting is that we may feel compassion for characters "displaying traits we would find unbearable or appalling in a real person" (John, 2016, p. 32, drawing on Robinson, 2005). John goes on to explain, "As readers of fiction, we can carry ourselves with less certainty about what we care about and can feel more free to consider alternatives and challenges to our interests than we ordinarily can" (2016, p. 33). Similarly Alan H. Goldman (2013) suggests that knowing that we are reading fiction may make us more apt to be empathetic because we are less suspicious of people's motives and do not feel obligated to act on their behalf. Herein lies an enormous potential for fiction to cultivate reflection and personal growth in readers. Although we come to care about characters in what I would say is a people-like way, there is a freedom readers experience with fiction that we don't have in real life—the characters are removed from us, and we do not have to talk to or deal with them. Therefore, we are free to relate to them differently from how we may relate to real people. Characters that represent types of real people and their experiences open readers up to caring about the kinds of people they may not be predisposed to care for. Fiction truly carries a unique potential to foster empathy.

What tools of literary writing contribute to how readers feel about characters? How do we cultivate these relationships between readers and characters?

Fiction differs from other forms in two ways that are central to the cultivation of empathy. First, we can enter into the intimate thoughts of characters—their internal dialogue or interiority. This access to what people are thinking and feeling builds a deep connection between readers and characters. Social fiction authors can deliberately link particular concepts or ideas with forms of emotional engagement through characters readers care about. Abbott writes, "There is no disputing the power and flexibility of fiction for conveying ideas and wedding them with deep feeling" (2008, p. 154). Second, fictional narratives are incomplete and leave space for the readers' interpretations and imagination. Said another way, there are interpretive gaps in fiction, often intentionally included by the authors (de Freitas, 2003). Readers fill in these gaps, and in doing so they may actively develop empathetic connections to the characters (and the kinds of people they represent). Furthermore, as we read fiction, we engage our imaginations. In her review of Holocaust fiction Ruth Franklin notes, "[An] act of imagination is an act of empathy" (2011, p. 15). Both interiority and interpretive gaps are elaborated in later chapters.

Forging Micro–Macro Connections

Fiction is uniquely well suited to crystallizing micro–macro connections. In other words, fiction can be used to show the relationship between individuals' lives and the larger cultural and institutional contexts in which we live. Many scholars aim to make these connections explicit. This is particularly true in sociology, where many are influenced by C. Wright Mills's (1959) concept of "the sociological imagination." For example, Watson's 2020 novel *Into the Sea* explicitly explores this fundamental concept, and in doing so weaves a sociological perspective throughout the entire narrative. For another example, public health researcher and sociologist Jessica Smartt Gullion's 2014 novel *October Birds* explores what might happen during a global pandemic (made all the more timely by recent events). In the fictional narrative Gullion links the experiences of individual characters to larger structural and policy issues related to public health and the role of first responders in a crisis.

The same literary tools that can be used to promote empathetic engagement can also assist writers in making micro–macro connections. For instance, interior dialogue can be used to show how something external impacts a character's thoughts and feelings. The subtext of my novel *Low-Fat Love* is about how toxic images and stories in popular culture may negatively influence women, resulting in low self-esteem, poor body image, and unhealthy relationship ideals. To illustrate the effect of commercial pop culture on women's lives, I often showed the protagonist consuming media (e.g., made-for-television movies, home shopping). During these scenes readers have access to her interiority—how what she watched made her feel.

Self and Social Reflection

All research is aimed at generating new insights, new learning. There are countless ways that fiction can teach, including providing information about historical or contemporary events. Perhaps more than anything else, the learning that happens with fiction results from gaining access to the different perspectives of the characters we come to care about or simply sympathize with. I believe the way readers develop new insights when reading fiction is through self and social reflection. As we read about characters and their stories, we may reflect on our own lives and the larger society. In this respect, fiction offers a way to challenge stereotypes.

How do we illuminate that which is taken for granted as "the way things are"? How can we challenge stereotypes? How do we get others to learn and care about different people, including those they may hold negative assumptions about? How might we disrupt dominant cultural narratives and myths, making room for new ways of thinking and seeing?

All the strengths of fiction discussed in this chapter foster the kind of reflection that has the ability to change individuals. By creating realistic story-worlds, readers may become immersed—ultimately exploring worlds that are similar and/or dissimilar to their own—seeing those worlds in new ways and through new eyes. Through empathetic engagement, which occurs as readers develop concern for characters that serve as guides in the story-world, we reflect on the situations the characters are in and, by extension, our own lives and the lives of others. As readers begin to care for the characters and develop empathy, previously held assumptions, values, and even worldviews can be challenged.

I can tell you that from the stories readers have shared with me over the years in response to my own works of fiction, I am certain this happens regularly as readers engage with fiction; it becomes a springboard for self and social reflection, increased awareness, and a reevaluation of previously held assumptions. However, if your own experiences reading fiction and my anecdotal evidence is not persuasive, there's actually quantitative research contending that fictional stories do change readers' beliefs. Deborah A. Prentice, Richard J. Gerrig, and Daniel S. Bailis (1997) conducted experimental research in which participants were given fictional narratives that contained weak or unsupported assertions. Although there were some mixed results, overall participants were influenced by and accepted the assertions. Wheeler et al. (1999) replicated the experiment. They did not have mixed results and found that participants were influenced by and accepted the assertions. They write:

> Across all three replications, we found that individuals were persuaded by story assertions. . . . The Prentice et al. experiments and our replications constitute strong evidence for the persuasiveness of narratives. (p. 140)

This research shows what many readers and writers of fiction already understand: fictional narratives can change readers' belief systems. Beliefs and values influence human action and are inextricably linked. So when we influence beliefs, we become a part of shaping what people think and therefore what they do. Imagine the potential social fiction has for sensitizing people to stereotypes, among other topics, and offering alternative ways to think, see, and feel.

If anyone ever says you cannot change the world through fiction, they are wrong. You can reshape yourself and others and in turn the larger environment in which we live. When we create possible worlds in fiction, we unleash the potential to remake our own.

Conclusion

Magic, inspiration, art, aesthetics, empathy, reflection—these are not ideas we often read about in research methods books. Yet they are a part of the research process, and they are certainly integral to writing and understanding social fiction. They in no way detract from the rigor and discipline needed to write social fiction. Creativity and discipline are not mutually exclusive. False polarizations have plagued academic research practice for far too long. Our research practice can be both fun and challenging. The writing we produce can be both engaging and informative. And writing fiction can be both scholarship and art.

Ultimately your writing practice is your own, as unique as your fingerprint. No two imaginations are alike, and how we take what we see in our mind's eye and translate that into pen on paper, is entirely original. No one can invent story-worlds as you might, so for those possible realities to exist, we need you to write them. The characters we as authors create come through our filters, and no one else could birth them. Yet they exist independently of us, their stories resonate with many, and their lessons are available to all. Our characters also reveal pieces of themselves through the creation process that we could not have anticipated. So while this book will give you the basic tools you need to develop a writing discipline, be on the lookout for magic. It's always right around the corner. Sometimes we can even catch it.

This book is an invitation. We can do research in literary ways. I hope the pages that follow encourage you to develop your own creative writing practice. The turn to social fiction is not a new invention. It is a re/invention. You can be a part of it. This book is also a road map. In the chapters that follow you'll be taken through the growing and shifting terrain of social fiction, through which there are innumerable paths. What paths will you create?

SKILL-BUILDING EXERCISE Select a general research topic using the strategies noted in this chapter. Develop writing prompts: quick sentences or phrases based on your topic. For example, if your topic is domestic violence, your prompts could be any of the following: he was in a rage again, she cowered in the corner, she threw their clothes into a garbage bag, or the shelter couldn't accommodate children. Select one of your prompts and free write for 20 minutes. Don't fret too much. Just write.

RETHINK YOUR RESEARCH Think about your research topic, research participants (or potential participants), the participants' primary setting, and the central ideas related to your topic. Imagine a fictional rendering based on these factors and free write for 20 minutes. Don't fret too much. Just write. If you're not sure where to begin, select a snippet of data (e.g., a phrase a participant said, a definition from the literature, a note about the setting) and use it as a jumping-off point.

2

Historical and Contemporary Context for Social Fiction

> *Humanity has but one product, and that is fiction.*
> —Annie Dillard

The work of researchers and novelists aren't as disparate as some may claim. On the contrary, there has always been a winding road between research practice and the writing of fiction (Franklin, 2011). Stephen Banks writes that "the zone between the practices of fiction writers and non-fiction writers is blurry," because fiction "is only more or less 'fictional'" (2008, pp. 155–156). Similarly, JT Torres (2021) writes that "it may not be possible to conceive of any kind of knowledge *outside* of fiction. The raw matter of experience at some point, in order to be shared, must be arranged and delivered in a particular way . . . all language is a narrative act."

While I've heard scholars suggest that the use of fiction in research is a relatively new practice, in actuality, there is a long, robust, and complex history of merging fiction and research or fiction and nonfiction. It's impossible to capture this history in full, but it's important to have some sense of the context for social fiction, so in this abridged review I consider historical uses of fiction in the social sciences and humanities (emphasizing philosophy), historical fiction, creative nonfiction, contemporary qualitative research (including narrative inquiry and narrative autoethnography), arts-based research, and literary neuroscience. Finally I review the role of the movement toward public scholarship across academia.

Fiction in the Humanities and Social Sciences

We know that many novelists explicitly bring social, cultural, political, and other concerns to their work. For example, well-known authors, including Toni Morrison, Amy Tan, Paulla Ebron, Anna Tsing, and Alice Walker, have brought social science concerns into the public domain through their literary works (Behar, 1995). The reverse happens too. Intellectuals have also long brought their scholarship into fruition via fiction. I would even go further and suggest that historically many of our leading thinkers and writers have simultaneously been scholars and novelists, and there's no value in trying to make a distinction. They are both at once.

The use of literary writing to unearth and communicate intellectual concerns perhaps began with philosophy, generally considered the oldest discipline and mother of all scholarly disciplines. It's no wonder there are countless academic books on philosophy and literature. Many scholars have devoted their professional lives to analyzing the relationship between philosophy and literature. Furthermore, there's a seemingly endless list of contemporary and older novels, plays, and short stories that explicitly address philosophical concerns. Rebecca Hussey (2021) offers a useful way to distinguish philosophical fiction from straight-up fiction, suggesting that "philosophical fiction deals with ideas in a direct way" and to a large degree, encouraging readers "to ponder big questions." In other words, it's purposeful in its intent to raise big ideas and prompt reader engagement with those ideas. This is exactly how I distinguished social fiction from generic fiction in the last chapter. It's about author expertise, perspective, and intent, which in turn affects the readers' experience. Hussey (2021) explains further:

> Sometimes this fiction contains actual philosophizing in it: characters might argue over ideas or a narrator might make a case for a certain way of looking at the world. Sometimes this fiction embodies ideas in its storytelling, so the philosophizing is implicit rather than explicit. Reading this type of philosophical fiction, we experience the ideas or viewpoint as we absorb the story.

Let's look at a couple of examples.

Jean-Paul Sartre is widely regarded as a leader of existentialist philosophy, much of which he communicated through literary art. For example, his play *No Exit* is an existential exploration. The story follows three characters in hell awaiting their fate, only to realize hell is one another. Sartre's novel *Nausea* presents an exploration of human consciousness and is considered a treatise on existentialism. Sartre's renowned body of philosophical work was largely presented through fictional works, such as plays and novels, including a trilogy. His inquiry *and* the representation of that inquiry are indeed fictional works. For those skeptical about the concept of "social fiction" bear in mind that Sartre won the Nobel Prize for his work (although he refused to accept it). His work is a shining example of the belief that philosophical or social fiction can communicate ideas purposefully *and* be good art, even exceptional art.

Simone de Beauvoir also produced great philosophical publications in both nonfiction and fictional formats, and received numerous honors for her work. Also considered a leading figure in existentialism, de Beauvoir developed a feminist existential position, exploring gender inequality and the potential to transcend such inequality. Her famed nonfiction book *The Second Sex* (published in 1949) explored how women are defined in relation to men. However, it is in her many compelling works of fiction that the processes by which this occurs and the effect on women's lives can best be felt and understood. For example, *The Woman Destroyed* is a set of three novellas (originally published in the 1960s): *The Age of Discretion, The Monologue,* and *The Woman Destroyed*. Each one is written using first-person narration from the perspective of the female protagonist, although different styles are employed: a scenic narrative, a monologue, and a series of chronological diary-style entries, respectively. Each story follows a middle-age or older woman facing a confluence of interrelated crises—the loss of passion with her male partner, infidelity, halted academic success, grown children who no longer "need" her. In each story, the narrator takes us on a journey through part of her life—the choices she made in the context of relationships to others—and what she has been left with as a result. We see the process that led her from point A to point B in her life, all through her own unfolding analysis and reflection.

I find *The Woman Destroyed,* the longest of the three novellas, the most compelling. The diary-style entries begin with the protagonist enjoying a trip to the countryside, musing about how wonderful life is. In the 125 pages that follow, we see her happiness diminish, her mind-set and life spiraling down a dark hole. Her beloved husband is having an affair. We are witness to her psychological process and how it unfolds over many months, from her initial thought that it's a meaningless, fleeting affair to her utter devastation that her husband is leaving her. As this process unravels, we bear witness to the choices she has made over the course of their relationship—her role as mother to two daughters, her focus on family over work life, her blind eye to infidelity, the changes in her own personality, which result from her role as wife and mother. By the end of the story, she is but a shell, frightened and alone. She writes: "Now I am a dead woman. A dead woman who still has years to drag out—how many?" (1969, p. 253). Her husband is gone. Her children are gone. She sits in her apartment looking at closed doors. She writes:

> The door to the future will open. Slowly. Unrelentingly. I am on the threshold. There is only this door and what is waiting behind it. I am afraid. And I cannot call to anyone for help. I am afraid. (1969, pp. 253–254)

In this fictional story, de Beauvoir examines the existential death of a woman, and shows readers in painstaking detail exactly how this death occurs in the context of a patriarchal society in which women's identities are relationally based. It is philosophy. It is theory. It is fiction. And it is powerful.

Fiction has also long been used by scholars outside of philosophy to address social and cultural issues. While Sartre and de Beauvoir were celebrated in their time, many other scholars have been met with scrutiny and critique, including those whose work has later been revered. Zora Neale Hurston is a clear example. It's also important to acknowledge that as a woman of color, the critiques leveled against her were particularly harsh.

Hurston, an anthropologist and author, published four novels and more than 50 short stories, plays, and essays, which center on the experiences of women of color. Due to mistreatment, she never completed her doctorate in anthropology and was subjected to repeated criticism at Columbia University for failing to conform to standards of "rigor" (Harrison, 1995; Visweswaran, 1994). It's now easy to understand that she was pushing her field forward, both in terms of content (writing about race and gender) and form (using literary writing). Today Hurston is widely considered an anthropological novelist. She went beyond the confines of traditional anthropology and decided to use literary tools to write "against the grain" of both the academy and the larger patriarchal, white supremacist culture (Behar, 1995; Harrison, 1995). In this way, Hurston's turn to fiction, specifically ethnographically informed fiction, allowed her to simultaneously challenge dominant understandings of race, class, and gender as well as the academic apparatus that excluded the resistive form and content of her work. Faye V. Harrison (1995) studied Hurston's work and contends:

> [Her] fiction was grounded in a contextual, participatory ethnographic subjectivity which during her lifetime had no comfortable home in American anthropology. . . . Hers is a holistic fiction that reflects her vision of a pluralistic yet human-centered set of interlocking experiences. Her creative work boldly envisions and interprets. (pp. 235, 241)

Hurston's powerful work is both aesthetically strong and culturally significant.

> The process of fictionalizing is impacted by gender, race, and other status characteristics. Fiction emerges through the filter of its author. While we often hear discussions of how these factors shape the work of women and those who identify as BIPOC (Black, indigenous, and people of color), it's true for all authors. Carefully consider your positionality and how it influences your experiences and perspectives on the world and your research. Consider how your identity positions you in relation to the stories you want to tell, how it shapes those stories, and what is your ethical responsibility to tell stories you are qualified to tell and to tell those stories sensitively.

The preceding works are merely examples. Countless lesser-known scholar-writers have approached their work in a similar fashion. In the discipline of history, fiction isn't even purported to be an aberration. Fiction has long been used as a means of addressing, analyzing, and presenting historical topics. The historical novel is so popular it's a genre in its own right.

Historical Fiction

Many of my loved ones enjoy reading historical novels as a means of being transported to another time or place, being exposed to other lifestyles and cultures, and learning about a different set of human experiences. They routinely tell me how much they learn from the novels they have read, and how enjoyable the learning experience is. Statements often begin with "I had no idea that . . . " and usually end with, "Did you know about that?" Often this reading experience not only teaches information but also fosters sympathetic or empathetic understanding by offering a picture of "what it was like" through characters the readers can identify with and/or come to care about. People report feeling a connection to individuals who are vastly different from themselves or who live in foreign places and situations. Chanel Cleeton (2021) explains, "Historical fiction has the unique ability to transport the reader back in time, to allow them to see historical events through the lens of characters that inhabit the story. Historical fiction empowers readers to look at history from a fresh perspective, and to traverse time periods, settings, and points of view you otherwise might not have been exposed to." It's not surprising that historical fiction often tackles social justice issues.

Historical fiction can serve as a way to get at issues of inequality—for example, what it means to be a woman, a person of color, an LGBTQIA individual, or an economically disadvantaged person in a specific time and place. In this way historical fiction can educate people, document the experience of disenfranchised groups, and build bridges across differences. The content of historical fiction often centers on a particularly challenging time or event and how people experienced it. In this regard, Holocaust fiction has become its own genre. I explore some of the history and debate surrounding Holocaust fiction because it powerfully reveals the key contested issues that emerge in historical fiction more broadly.

Ruth Franklin (2011) chronicled the emergence and impact of Holocaust fiction in her book *A Thousand Darknesses: Lies and Truth in Holocaust Fiction*. Testimonial memoirs are the primary form Holocaust writing takes. Many scholars have argued that firsthand accounts are the only responsible way to represent the event. This argument is guided by two beliefs: (1) The Holocaust is such a unique event that it is not knowable or accessible and can only be preserved via firsthand accounts and (2) Not only is the Holocaust unspeakable, but it is also immoral to use such a horrific event as the material for fiction (Franklin, 2011). Lawrence Langer argued that it is unethical to turn the suffering of genocide victims into art for "the world that murdered them" (Franklin, 2011, p. 5). This stance recalls the famous quote by Theodor Adorno: "To write a poem after Auschwitz is barbaric." Whereas this statement has been interpreted in different ways, most suggest it is "a condemnation of the moral callousness of aestheticizing horror" (Franklin, 2011, p. 2).

For others who welcome the use of fiction to represent the Holocaust, the response to the preceding arguments is twofold. First many scholars take issue with the assumption that diaries and testimonials are pure nonfiction. In what form would they have to be archived or published in order to qualify as pure? For example, Anne Frank's diary, one of the most well-known pieces of Holocaust writing, was edited or "cleaned up" by her father prior to publication. Different versions of the diary, including some aimed at children, have been subsequently published. But even when the texts we read are the original ones, their authors have been engaging in a narrative process that involves the selection of themes and details. James Edward Young (cited in Franklin, 2011) notes that all diaries and testimonials contain narratives and thus merge nonfiction and fiction. Similarly Franklin writes: "Every act of memory is also an act of narrative" (2011, p. 12).

A second argument made by those who support the use of fiction to represent the Holocaust is that through art we are better able to enter into and understand this "unimaginable" event—fiction allows us to imagine. It is this response that best aligns with the principles of this book. It is also here that we see the greatest fear that Holocaust fiction evokes: "a more general anxiety about the ways in which we respond to and value art and the uses to which we are prepared to put it" (Franklin, 2011, p. 5). Traces of this fear underscore many debates in the research community when fiction and nonfiction are overtly blurred.

It is important to consider carefully the benefits that some attribute to fictionalized representations of the Holocaust, since through them we can appreciate the potential of social fiction across the disciplines. There are three primary reader experiences Holocaust fiction can evoke: understanding, imagination, and empathy. They are all interconnected and are vital if we are to learn compassionately from this past horror.

How do you help people to make sense of historical events, particularly those that seem beyond understanding? Jorge Semprun suggests that understanding is a function of effective storytelling, and that this can't be done well without some artifice—"enough to make it art" (Franklin, 2011, p. 13). Meaningful understanding also requires imagination. For example, often when people watch a film about a historical event or time period, whether it is the Holocaust, the slave trade, the September 11 attacks, the attack on Pearl Harbor, or the sinking of the Titanic, they imagine what the experience was like, who they would have been in that time and place, and how they would have acted and reacted to the larger sociohistorical forces at work. All of this imagining is an integral part of the process of learning. Franklin writes, "We need literature about the Holocaust not only because testimony is inevitably incomplete, but because of what literature uniquely offers: an imaginative access to past events, together with new and different ways of understanding them that are unavailable to strictly factual forms of writing" (2011, p. 13). It is through the process of imaginatively putting ourselves in the shoes of others that we are able to develop compassion and empathy. Through fictional accounts we can learn from history in order to avoid repeating it.

Despite some resistance, the common wisdom seems to be that fiction can help us understand history. Therefore, a plethora of novels, plays, and films about the Holocaust have been produced. What many have learned about the Holocaust and felt in response to this event comes from these artistic renderings. Some argue that the continued production of these representations points to a "cultural hunger for novels, films, plays" (Franklin, 2011, p. 5) because they can help us understand and bear witness.

In 1946, what is widely considered the first Holocaust novel, *Sunrise over Hell*, was published in Israel. The novel was authored by Ka-Tzetnik 135633, which translates to "Concentration camp inmate 135633." This early novel shows that fictional formats were a part of Holocaust writing from the very beginning. For a more recent example of blurring within the genre of Holocaust representations, consider the book *Schindler's List* (1982) by Thomas Keneally. Many know the book through Steven Spielberg's (1993) award-winning film adaptation. Interestingly Keneally termed his book a nonfiction novel, pointing to the inevitable blurring of fiction and nonfiction in Holocaust literature. Or consider the 2006 novel *The Boy in the Striped Pajamas* by the Irish novelist John Boyne, which was released as a film in 2008.

The tradition of Holocaust fiction has continued with other events (for example, the Rwandan genocide and the Bosnian War). In recent years there has also been an increase in fiction depicting the Israeli–Palestinian conflict. This conflict is one of the most important, complex, and divisive human rights issues of our time. Here fiction may be particularly useful since it offers the ability to develop empathy and compassion as we become aware of others' experiences and perspectives in a disarming way.

Before discussing the contemporary academy and the role of qualitative and ABR in setting the stage for social fiction, it's worthwhile to briefly consider how the emergence of creative nonfiction in the media influenced the turn to narrative. The academy does not exist in a vacuum.

Creative Nonfiction

Creative nonfiction arose in the 1960s and 1970s as a means of making research reports more engaging while remaining truthful (Caulley, 2008; Goodall, 2008). In the commercial world of trade publishing and journalism as well as in academic writing and publishing, writers were looking for ways to use literary tools in order to strengthen their factual writing. Lee Gutkind, founder of *Creative Nonfiction* magazine, proclaims creative nonfiction to be the fastest-growing genre in publishing, and says that at its core the genre promotes "true stories well told" (2012). He further defines the form as follows:

> The word "creative" refers to the use of literary craft, the techniques fiction writers, playwrights, and poets employ to present nonfiction—factually accurate prose about real people and events—in a compelling, vivid, dramatic manner. The goal is to make nonfiction stories read like fiction so that your readers are as enthralled by fact as they are by fantasy. But the stories are true. (p. 6)

The commercialization of newspaper reporting has normalized the tenets of creative nonfiction within the public sphere. Norms in academic writing have changed as a result. If once-purported "objective" journalists could actively engage in crafting good stories by adapting literary techniques, then academic researchers were emboldened to do the same. Moreover, as readers have become more accustomed to reading *stories* rather than *reports,* expectations have changed, opening up the possibilities for academic writers. The rise of creative nonfiction has put a premium on good storytelling. For many it isn't enough for research to "report" or "chronicle" events, but it should also do it well. This requires literary artifice. When stories are expressed well, readers are more deeply affected. Theodore A. Rees Cheney (2001) describes creative nonfiction as follows:

> Creative nonfiction tells a story using facts, but uses many of the techniques of fiction for its compelling qualities and emotional vibrancy. Creative nonfiction doesn't just report facts, it delivers facts in ways that move the reader toward a deeper understanding of a topic. Creative nonfiction requires the skills of the storyteller and the research ability of the conscientious reporter. (p. 1)

It's worth remembering that although using literary techniques in order to make stories engaging has become a norm in journalism, creative nonfiction in this arena is intended to remain strictly factual. Recently *Der Spiegel*, a top German news magazine, made international headlines when it was discovered that star reporter and editor Claas Relotius had falsified articles, fabricating facts and sources. Relotius was forced to resign. The slope of what's acceptable is more slippery in academia, depending on the method used and the disclosures made about creating composite characters or other means of fictionalizing.

In academia, researchers are storytellers, learning about others and sharing what they have learned. Whether we go into the field in an ethnographic study or conduct oral history interviews, we are charged with telling the stories of others in creative, expressive, dynamic, and authentic ways. We may also be relying on our own autoethnographic experiences as data that explicitly informs the stories we craft. Bud Goodall termed this "the new ethnography" (2000, 2008). When we represent and share our research, our goal is not simply to expose others to it, but to *affect* those who read our work. The goals of particular projects—educating, raising awareness, exposing myths, building critical consciousness, disrupting dominant ideologies or stereotypes, putting a human face on an issue, and so on—may vary, but whatever our objective, we aim to affect our readers. Just like with good teaching, we hope our research is written well enough to make a lasting impact. Well-written stories are memorable.

Creative nonfiction is an expansive genre. Research articles, essays, op-eds, blogs, and books may all be written in this fashion and commonly are. Laurel Richardson has long been an inspirational figure to those writing in these new shapes. While she has called her work "writing-stories" and experimental writing, Tom Barone (2008) perceptively noted that her groundbreaking book *Fields of Play* can be considered creative nonfiction. Another example that is routinely cited in the research community is Truman Capote's *In Cold Blood* (1966), which some suggest can be considered a qualitative research project

> In order to avoid any confusion or accusations of wrongdoing, if you choose to present your fiction as research or research as fiction, be up-front and honest. Disclose the creative liberties taken, the fictitious elements, and the role of the imaginative in the final work.

because of the copious research the author conducted (Norris, 2009). In sum creative nonfiction, within and beyond the academy, has changed how many view academic writing and has brought the tools of literary fiction into the researcher's purview.

Qualitative Research

Let's turn to inside the contemporary academy. Using fiction as a social research practice is a natural extension of what many researchers and writers have long been doing. Fiction writers, like social scientists, conduct extensive research to achieve verisimilitude (Banks, 2008; Berger, 1977). As noted in Chapter 1, verisimilitude refers to the creation of a realistic, authentic, and lifelike portrayal, and it is the goal of both fiction and established social science practices including ethnography. Fiction writers and qualitative researchers both seek to build believable representations of existing or possible worlds (Visweswaran, 1994, p. 1) and to portray human experience truthfully and authentically. It is not as if fiction writers *create* fantasies and researchers *record* facts. The material writers use in fiction is derived from real life and genuine human experience. Similarly, qualitative researchers very much shape every aspect of their investigation, imbuing it with meaning and marking it with their fingerprint.

Social research is a process aimed at knowledge building and meaning-making; at accessing, expressing, and negotiating contextual truths; and then at effectively communicating those "truths" to relevant audiences. Characterized as a craft, qualitative research aims to generate deep understanding, unpack meanings, reveal social processes, and above all illuminate human experience. Qualitative research values sensory knowledge and experience, multiple meanings, and subjectivity in the research process. In recent years, many qualitative practitioners have reconceptualized the researcher's role in ethnographic studies and the way to best represent that research. Reflexive writing is increasingly common, which Elizabeth de Freitas defines as writing that "traces the presence of the author in/through the text" (2007, p. 1).

There are a couple of contemporary qualitative research methods that especially relate to social fiction: narrative inquiry and narrative autoethnography.

Narrative Inquiry

Methods that draw on narrative writing exist on a science–art continuum. Some approaches to narrative inquiry are closer to traditional qualitative research practice, particularly interview research, whereas others are closer to the artistic side and draw significantly on literary traditions. Mark Freeman (2007) has rightfully suggested that artful approaches to narrative inquiry can contribute to ethical practice by increasing sympathy and compassion (p. 142). Candace Stout (2014) has explored the bonds between narrative art and narrative inquiry as a means of calling forth the "centers" or resonant cores of stories. Bochner and Herrmann (2020) suggest that narrative inquiry exists somewhere between art and science.

Writing is, and has always been, an integral part of research practice. Researchers use language or "the word" as a communicative device employed in the service of social scientific knowledge building. All research, regardless of paradigm, involves writing. Narratives—or stories about something (Labov, 2006)—have also long been a part of research practice.[1] There is a rich tradition of storytelling methods in the qualitative paradigm that draw on cultural practices of oral knowledge transmission, such as oral history and life history.

Researchers who use narrative do so for many reasons and in a variety of ways. They tend to have a common desire to breathe humanity into their work and to tell stories (their own and those of others) in more truthful, engaged, and resonant ways and a desire to do work that has the potential to increase connectivity and reflection. Many wish to engage more collaboratively with their participants and ultimately produce work that can be read by many. Narrative researchers attempt to avoid the objectification of research participants and aim to preserve the complexity of human experience (Josselson, 2006). Bochner and Herrmann (2020) view narrative inquiry as a way to "humanize the human sciences."

Narrative inquiry builds on the tenets of ethnography and oral history in order to collaboratively unearth participants' life experiences and engage in a process of storying and re-storying. Narratives are constructed out of the data through a reflexive, participatory, and aesthetic process. In a narrative method, data are analyzed using narrative analysis or a "narrative mode of analysis" (Kim, 2015, p. 197). Jeong-Hee Kim explains that narrative analysis is a process whereby "the researcher extracts an emerging theme from the fullness of lived experiences presented in the data themselves and configures stories making a range of disconnected research elements coherent, so that the story can appeal to the reader's understanding and imagination" (2006, p. 5).

Mary R. Harvey, Elliot G. Mishler, Karestan Koenan, and Patricia A. Harney (2000) identify three major components of narratives: coherence, turning points, and re-plotting.

Coherence refers to how a narrative is communicated or how the story hangs together. We may assume that research participants share cohesive or coherent narratives; however, this is often not the case, particularly when there has been trauma (Harvey et al., 2000, p. 295). For example, an initial story may be relayed episodically or in a fragmented manner, and later re-storied, ultimately producing a cohesive narrative. Turning points are often vital to participants' structuring of their narratives and the experiences to which they attest. They generally represent a shift in experience or interpretation. Re-plotting or re-storying is a primary aspect of narrative research. This is a process whereby participants narrativize their stories through the interplay between available cultural frames and individual meaning, which changes over time (Harvey et al., 2000, p. 307). In addition, re-storying occurs over time, as participants reflect on their own major life experiences and reframe them.

Although narrative inquiry is a collaborative qualitative research practice and differs significantly from writing fiction, it is in many ways a precursor to contemporary practices of writing social fiction. Moreover, the features of narratives reviewed bear similarities that are pertinent to writing fictional narratives. Fiction writers aim to produce cohesive narratives, which is a benchmark upon which our work may be evaluated. These narratives often involve rising action, inciting incidents, and resolution, all of which have similarities to "turning points" (and are reviewed in detail in Chapter 4). Finally, through our pens, characters replot their own stories—they may change course, evolve, or be redeemed. They wind up different from how they began.

Narrative Autoethnography

Autoethnography is a method whereby researchers use their personal experience as a means of connecting the personal to a larger cultural context or phenomenon (Adams, Holman Jones, & Ellis, 2015). In other words, autoethnography values the researcher's personal experiences as a way of studying and writing about culture. There are many approaches to autoethnography (see Holman Jones, Adams, & Ellis, 2013), but for the sake of this discussion I focus on narrative autoethnography, which is traditional autoethnographic writing that is represented as a narrative or story. Narrative autoethnography exists on a continuum, beginning with researchers sharing personal experiences with their participants, which then become part of the larger research narrative, to wholly autobiographical projects, to those that explicitly combine autobiographical data and fiction. In all instances, this writing is not merely about the self (as with autobiography), but rather a way of writing about the culture, using the self as a starting point for inquiry. As we write about ourselves, we learn about the larger context in which we live our lives. Our stories are nested within larger cultural stories. Carolyn Ellis (2004) pioneered autoethnography and defines this method as follows:

> "What is autoethnography?" you might ask. My brief answer: research, writing, story, and method that connect the autobiographical and personal to the cultural, social, and political. Autoethnographic forms feature concrete action, emotion, embodiment, self-consciousness, and introspection portrayed in dialogue, scenes, characterization, and plot. Thus, autoethnography claims the conventions of literary writing. (p. xix)

This practice combines autobiographical writing with the conventions of narrative writing, often incorporating fiction (although certainly not always). Autoethnography may be communicated as a short story, essay, blog, vlog, poem, novel, play, performance piece, or other artful text. Researchers may fictionalize aspects of the work in order to create characterizations (which may be composites) as a means of situating the piece within a particular cultural and historical context to evoke mood or emotionality or to follow plot conventions. In autoethnographic writing, fiction may therefore be employed as a means of emphasizing contextual and partial truths, revealing social meanings, and linking the experiences of individuals to the larger cultural and institutional context in which they live. This form of writing can therefore help researchers bridge the micro and macro levels of analysis and highlight particular aspects of their work (such as subjugated voices).

A primary advantage of this method is the possibility it has to raise self-consciousness and thereby promote reflexivity. However, placing oneself at the center of the research process carries its own set of considerations and burdens. Autoethnography requires researchers to make themselves vulnerable. You cannot predict the emotions you will experience throughout this process. In addition, by opening up their personal life to the public, a researcher lets go of some privacies and invites possible criticism. Some think of autoethnography as "writing on the edge—and without a safety net" (Vickers, 2002, p. 608). This can be painful. It may be helpful to have a support team in place to offer feedback throughout the process (Tenni, Smyth, & Boucher, 2003).

Narrative autoethnography also problematizes the insider–outsider dichotomy that guides some conventional qualitative research practice. It is important to note that narrative autoethnography revolves around writing and the written word more so than methods, such as interviewing and field research, which rely heavily on verbal communication and visual observations. In the case of autoethnographic narratives the researcher is writing, not speaking—an entirely different process (e.g., most people can speak more quickly than they can write, and you can revise what you write) (Hesse-Biber & Leavy, 2005, 2011; Maines, 2001). This is a clear example of a qualitative research method that is based primarily on writing. So while it differs significantly from social fiction, there are similarities as well.

Contemporary qualitative practices, including those that explicitly rely on narrative, helped pave the way for ABR, including the method of social fiction.

Arts-Based Research

Both the practice of qualitative research and artistic practice can be viewed as crafts. Qualitative researchers do not simply gather and write; they *compose, orchestrate,* and *weave* (Leavy, 2009, 2015, 2020b). As Valerie J. Janesick (2001) notes, the researcher is the instrument in qualitative research as in artistic practice. Moreover, both practices are holistic and dynamic, involving reflection, description, problem formulation and solving, and the ability to identify and explain intuition and creativity in the research process. Therefore, Janesick refers to qualitative researchers as "artist-scientists."

A major shift in academic research began in the 1970s, and by the 1990s arts-based practices constituted a new methodological genre (Sinner, Leggo, Irwin, Gouzouasis, & Grauer, 2006, p. 1226). Some suggest, as I do, that ABR constitutes a new paradigm. For example, ABR pioneer Shaun McNiff views art as a unique "transdisciplinary way of knowing and communicating" (2018, p. 24). What is ABR? Its practices are a set of methodological tools used by researchers across the disciplines during any or all phases of research, including data generation, analysis, interpretation, and representation. These emerging tools adapt the tenets of the creative arts in order to address research questions in holistic and engaged ways in which theory and practice are intertwined. In other words, in ABR, the arts are used as a part or all of the inquiry process. Arts-based practices draw on literary writing, music, dance, performance, visual art, film, and other mediums.

Arts-based practices have posed serious challenges to methods conventions, thus unsettling many assumptions about what constitutes research and knowledge. Eisner articulated the fear experienced by some as the methods borders are pushed, making way for artistic representation: "We have . . . concretized our view of what it means to know. We prefer our knowledge solid and like our data hard. It makes for a firm foundation, a secure place on which to stand. Knowledge as a process, a temporary state, is scary to many" (1997, p. 7). Despite the fears, ABR has taken off, especially over the last 15 years, because many scholars recognize its enormous potential for creating knowledge about the social world.

Intuitively many people realize that the arts can be a profound source of learning and thus useful for conducting research and communicating research findings. Both philosophy and science support these assumptions.

In their groundbreaking work, George Lakoff and Mark Johnson (1980) suggested that metaphor is not characteristic only of language, but it also is pervasive in human thought and action. They explained that our conceptual system is fundamentally metaphorical, which implies that "what we experience, and what we do every day is very much a matter of metaphor" (p. 3). Their work has clear implications for how we best reach and engage audiences with research.

Mark Turner's renowned book *The Literary Mind: The Origins of Thought and Language* (1996) argued that the common perception that the everyday mind is nonliterary and that the literary mind is optional is untrue. Turner believed that "the literary mind is the fundamental mind," and observed, "Story is a basic principle of mind. Most of our experience, our knowledge, and our thinking is organized as stories. The mental scope of story is magnified by projection—one-story helps us make sense of another. The projection of one-story onto another is parable" (p. v).

For those for whom philosophical work isn't convincing, there's also "hard science" that shows we experience art—and literature in particular—differently from nonfiction prose.

Literary Neuroscience

When you're deep into a novel you're reading, you may feel like the house could burn down and you wouldn't notice because you're completely immersed. There's actually a physiological explanation for this common experience. Research in neuroscience, cognitive science, and psychology suggests that we become more engaged in reading fiction than nonfiction prose, and the effects can last longer. It's important to note that research consistently shows these effects occur as a result of close or "deep" reading (Paul, 2013). In other words, our brains become increasingly activated when we engage in deep reading that is immersive, in contrast with the quick scroll-style reading we may do on the Internet as we zip through stories (Paul, 2013). Psychologist Victor Nell (1988) studied what occurs when people read for pleasure, and found that they slow their pace. This kind of close, careful reading leads to deeper immersion and reflection. In later parts of this book when I encourage you to make your writing as strong as you can—to make it good art—bear in mind that readers must enjoy a work of fiction in order to have this type of immersive, reflective experience.

"Literary neuroscience" explores how different forms of reading affect brain activity.[2] For example, Natalie Phillips became interested in studying distractibility. She said: "I love reading, and I am someone who can actually become so absorbed in a novel that I really think the house could possibly burn down around me and I wouldn't notice. And I'm simultaneously someone who loses their keys at least three times a day, and I often can't remember where in the world I parked my car" (quoted in Thompson & Vedantam, 2012). Phillips and her research team conducted a study measuring brain activity as research participants engaged in close versus casual reading of a Jane Austen novel. They have found that the whole brain appears to be transformed as people engage in close readings of fiction. There are global activations across a number of different regions of the brain, including in some unexpected areas, such as those that are involved in movement and touch. In the experiment, it was as if "readers were physically placing themselves within the story as they analyzed it" (Thompson & Vedantam, 2012). Similarly Gregory Berns led a team of researchers in a study published in *Brain Connectivity* that suggests there is heightened connectivity in our brains for days after reading a novel (Berns, Blaine, Prietula, & Pye, 2013).

> In order to understand how to write fiction, it's important to understand the experience of reading fiction. Do a little experiment on yourself. Read a novel by one of your favorite writers or something you're simply bursting to read. Monitor your own reading experience. Notice your pace as you read. Observe whether your awareness of time passing changes. When you put the book down, do you find yourself thinking about it? When you finish it, does it linger? If so, what does it make you reflect on?

So what does it matter that our brains are transformed through closely reading fiction? What does reader immersion into story-worlds mean for researchers wishing to write social fiction? In the last chapter I said that the strengths of social fiction include sensitively portraying lived experience, achieving verisimilitude, building empathetic understanding, forging micro–macro connections, promoting self and social reflection, and challenging stereotypes. How are those ends achieved? They result from the process that occurs when readers become engaged in what they're reading—immersed in the story-world and invested in the characters who populate that reality. As authors of social fiction, we are creating those worlds and characters. Therefore, we can plant the seeds for reflection, new learning, and transformation. Annie Murphy Paul (2013) writes:

> That immersion is supported by the way the brain handles language in rich detail, allusion and metaphor: by creating a mental representation that draws on the same brain regions that would be active if the scene were unfolding in real life. The emotional situations and moral dilemmas that are the stuff of literature are also vigorous exercise for the brain, propelling us inside the heads of fictional characters and even, studies suggest, increasing our real-life capacity for empathy.

Fiction holds enormous promise for building sympathetic or empathetic understanding, which is the cornerstone of justice work and much contemporary research. When people casually say that they get lost in a good novel, that they imagine things about their favorite characters or feel as if they're friends, or simply that they love reading fiction, understand that these statements are profoundly meaningful. There is enormous and multifaceted pleasure to be found in reading. Wendy Lesser (2014) details this well in her book *Why I Read: The Serious Pleasure of Books*. The pleasure to be found in reading, which is intricately bound up with the way in which we read, offers perhaps unparalleled potential for researchers wishing to make meaningful and lasting impressions with their work. So as you embark on writing social fiction, if you face resistance from those in the academy who label it "soft," tell them "hard science" suggests otherwise. So does common sense.

Public Scholarship

Up to this point in this chapter I've addressed the historical uses of fiction in scholarly work as well as contemporary changes outside and inside the academy that have placed a premium on narratives in research. Perhaps the latest boon to social fiction results from the widespread effort to popularize scholarly research.

In recent years there has been a push for public scholarship, that is, scholarship that is accessible outside of the academy. The move to popularize research has made scholars reconsider the outcomes of their work and has led to many new ways of conducting and representing research, including the increased use of fiction as a research practice. Whereas traditional academic scholarship is inaccessible to the public, fiction can be read by virtually anyone. People elect to read fiction in their leisure time. Furthermore, when properly targeted to the stakeholders we aim to reach, for example, based on age, it can be crafted to suit those particular audiences. So for instance, research conducted about teenagers could actually reach teenagers (e.g., through a YA novel). Talk about a novel idea!

Increasingly people view research that is inaccessible to public audiences and disconnected from public needs to be of little value. Although public scholarship has always existed and been a regular part of the academic and/or public discourse since the 1960s (Denzin & Giardina, 2018), it has gained considerable attention over the past two decades. Many inside and outside of the academy have critiqued traditional research practices for resulting in a wellspring of research that circulates exclusively within the academy and garners a shockingly small readership even within that elite sphere. Some studies have shown that most academic journal articles have as few as three to eight readers. So the idea that peer-reviewed journal articles are even well read in the academy has long been seriously overestimated.

The small audience for journal articles is easy to explain. Peer-reviewed articles are inaccessible in two key ways. First, they circulate in hard-to-get journals that are available in university libraries. Few people are aware of these journals or have reasonable and affordable access to them. Second, academic journal articles are loaded with discipline-specific jargon. They're difficult to understand and generally fail to meet the standards of good and engaging writing, certainly from a literary point of view. They're dense and boring. There, I said it.

In 2014 former *New York Times* columnist Nicholas Kristof wrote a scathing indictment of the academic research system, noting that professors, although among the most knowledgeable people, have made themselves irrelevant in conversations of import. He contends that it isn't merely that they've been marginalized, but also that they have "marginalized themselves." Kristof likens academic writing to "gobbledygook" that is often "hidden in obscure journals." As Kristof suggests, this is bigger than individual academic researchers who are simply trying to get jobs and earn tenure and promotion, but is rather a product of an arcane professional system in desperate need of updating.

So what is public scholarship? Most simply, public scholarship is that which is available outside of the academy. Lay citizens have access to public scholarship in two areas: it circulates in spaces to which they have access *and* it's understandable (Leavy, 2011, 2019a, 2021a, 2021b, 2021c).

Public scholarship has always existed, to some extent, but has become the focus of debate over the past 25 years. Michael Burawoy's 2004 American Sociological Association Presidential Address, devoted to public sociology, is frequently credited as a turning point. While this event certainly is a noteworthy moment in the historical time line, it is also a problematic one for two key reasons. First, many sociologists have long engaged in this kind of work, whether or not they were properly recognized in the academic reward and "fame" structure that itself is highly hierarchical and insular. For example, Patricia Hill Collins explains that before the term "public sociology" was popularized, she was long "doing a kind of sociology that had no name" (2007, p. 101). Collins ultimately earned rock star status in academia, but most do not, and carry on with this work in the shadows. Even those who have done this work and received recognition are operating from the margins, not from the center of the discipline (Collins, 2007). Second, as Evelyn Nakano Glenn has astutely pointed out, Burawoy's "social position" as a white male at an elite university permeated his conception of public sociology and the confidence with which he in fact mapped out the entire discipline of sociology in his speech (2007, p. 215).

The push toward public scholarship has been particularly strong in my home discipline of sociology. Many have taken Burawoy's call seriously and began to consider the "multiple publics" sociologists ought to reach and the "multiple ways" we might do so (Burawoy, 2005, p. 7). Fiction is one method sociologists have begun using to do so. As Watson writes, "Sociological novel writing can work to reconceptualise the traditional academic-audience relationship . . . positioning sociologists as writers, publics as readers, and both parties as interlocutors" (2016, p. 5). The power of fiction for sociologists in particular is, in part, that we can take "the immediate and everyday experiences of a public and hold it under a microscope: question values, challenge social processes, and create dissonance within the public's image of itself" (Watson, 2016, p. 6). Additionally, as I have written about in the past, fiction allows writers to flesh out micro–macro connections (see Leavy, 2013, 2015). Writers can show the relationship between an individual's personal biography and the larger social and historical contexts in which they live, a long-held goal of sociology thanks to C. Wright Mills, as noted in Chapter 1.

I should note that while the trend has increased over the past couple decades, sociologists also have a history of using fiction. Famed sociologist Lewis A. Coser was far ahead of his peers, when he published *Sociology through Literature: An Introductory Reader* in 1963. At the time he deemed the book experimental but believed that novelists were uniquely able to tap into and describe human experience, which could be of great value for teaching in the social sciences. There are many earlier works in literary criticism that also explore similar issues; for example, *Literature and Society* by David Daiches, which was published in 1938, and *The Truths of Fiction* by Allan Rodway, first published in 1958.

Challenges of Doing Fiction as Research

Despite the long history of social fiction in different fields and its increased use today, it's important to understand that there can be tremendous challenges in doing this work. These challenges are heightened for students and early-career researchers. For example, doing this kind of work as a masters thesis or doctoral dissertation, or as your publishing work before tenure and promotion, may be difficult. Many scholars are simply unfamiliar with social fiction or ABR more generally. Among those who are familiar, some do not view it as a legitimate method of inquiry. Therefore, satisfying thesis or tenure committees may be difficult. Even convincing your advisor that this is a valid form of research may be challenging. I absolutely understand these pragmatic concerns. The ability to graduate, secure a job, and earn promotion are major goals in a person's life that carry massive material and other consequences. I in no way wish to diminish that reality. Rather I encourage you to find ways to carve your own path through academia, doing work that is meaningful to you. I've written this chapter in part to arm you with information that will help you bolster and contextualize your work for gatekeepers who may be unfamiliar or uncomfortable with social fiction. Understand that by wanting to engage in this work you are in good company. Here are some practical strategies for dealing with barriers to doing this kind of work:

- When explaining your work to your professors or senior colleagues, avoid being defensive, and instead try to educate them about this kind of work. Point out some of the famous scholars who have used social fiction and that you are writing in their tradition.

- Use the citation system to bolster your work—cite the many scholars, past and present, who have used fiction in a similar way. You can also refer to scholars who have done other kinds of ABR on your specific topic area.

- Seek out external reviewers (for your thesis or tenure committee) who are familiar with social fiction or related methods.

- Attend conferences where ABR is valued and/or join online social media communities centered on ABR, on emergent or critical approaches to qualitative research, and on fiction or other creative writing. In doing so, develop a network of other folks doing similar work.

- Add nonfiction prose components to your work to satisfy review committees. For example, add a preface or afterword to your fictional works in which you explain your research.

- Publish your work in more than one form. For example, if you publish a short story or novel, consider writing a peer-reviewed article for a qualitative methods journal about your methodology and how it aided your project.

Conclusion

As scholars seek ways to make their work accessible, relevant, and engaging, fiction has emerged as a legitimate avenue for doing so. As we can see from looking at the work of some of our most revered philosophers, this is not so much a new method of inquiry, but rather a return to and evolution of an esteemed approach to scholarship and artistry. We're not inventing the wheel, simply pushing it forward. This is a re/invention. Social fiction has deep roots in numerous disciplines and yet transcends them all. It has been effectively used to stage epistemological debates and recount the struggles of daily life for people differently situated in the social order and so much more. The potential for social fiction to produce meaningful scholarship is limitless. And its illustrious history shows it should be taken seriously.

> **SKILL-BUILDING EXERCISE** Select and read a work of philosophical or historical fiction (e.g., a short story, play, novella, or novel). Write a one- to two-page response addressing what you have learned about the topic from the fictional work. Consider these questions: What ideas or historical events are central? How are they presented? What questions are posed? What did you learn? What, if any, new insights did you glean?

> **RETHINK YOUR RESEARCH** Select and read a popular or scholarly work of fiction centered on the topic of your research. Imagine your research participants as characters in the work, and imagine yourself as a character or the narrator. The goal is simply to start envisioning how your project could be reimagined into the story-world.

NOTES

1. Methods that expressly use narrative have been on the rise for over half a century. D. Jean Clandinin and Jerry Rosiek (2007) note that since the late 1960s narrative inquiry has become increasingly common across the disciplines. Bochner and Riggs (2014) detail the surge in narrative inquiry across different disciplines in the 1980s through the end of the 20th century, by which point the use of narrative intensified. They note the publication of Donald Spence's (1984) *Narrative Truths and Historical Truths* and Theodore Sarbin's (1986) edited volume *Narrative Psychology* as key

moments in the rise of the narrative in psychology, the most resistant of the social sciences. By the start of the 21st century the "narrative turn" had occurred (Bochner & Herrmann, 2020; Bochner & Riggs, 2014; Denzin & Lincoln, 2000). Bochner and Riggs (2014) point to an increase in personal narrative, life histories, life stories, testimonials, and memoirs as evidence of the widespread use of narrative across the social sciences.

2. It is interesting to note that the history of neuroscience itself is intertwined with fiction. Silas Weir Mitchell (1824–1914) is considered the father of American neurology (Todman, 2007). Interestingly he was also a fiction writer who published an astonishing 19 novels, 7 poetry books, and many short stories. Many of his works of fiction were inextricably bound to patient observations made during his clinical practice and centered on topics dealing with psychological and physiological crises. Given Mitchell's extensive body of fictional work, some suggest that students can learn about the history of neuroscience itself through his fictional writings (De Jong, 1982; Todman, 2007). Similarly, Charlotte Perkins Gilman's 1892 short story *The Yellow Wallpaper* is used in some neurology and neuroscience programs in order to illustrate concepts in mental illness and doctor–patient relationships with respect to sociohistorical and cultural understandings of gender (Todman, 2007).

3 The Method

How to Write Social Fiction

> Every story, every incident, every bit of conversation is raw material for me.
> —Sylvia Plath

You want to write fiction, but where do you begin? The truth is that the seeds of inspiration come to us in many ways. As I noted in Chapter 1, my own works of fiction have taken shape in different ways. Sometimes there's a theme or concept I want to explore, at other times I have the structure for a narrative and need to figure out the content, or a character takes shape in my mind, or a whole story comes to me in a burst and then I need to do the work to translate it. The truth is, it never happens the same way twice. That's part of the magic of writing fiction and why I'm still in love with it. Just as inspiration takes different forms, so too the writing process is never quite the same. In my own work, I've either written detailed outlines and then plodded away, chronologically writing the story, or I've just sat down and begun to write scenes totally out of order and later stitched them together. One of my novels was written in 10 days. There's another one I've been working on for nearly 10 years. Like I said, it rarely happens the same way twice. The more discipline and skill you develop around your writing practice, the more you'll be able to translate inspiration when it comes to you and the more you'll be able to broaden the ways in which you write.

The practice of writing social fiction is not a linear methodology. There is no one way to do it, no set of procedures that can simply be followed. The fact is that the writing process itself is a generative act—an act of discovery—and so no matter your approach to it, there are things you simply can't plan in advance. Those are actually the best parts. While there is no cookie-cutter model for how to write social fiction, consider using the narrative features and writing strategies that are reviewed in this chapter. Please don't take my suggestions as "the" way one must write social fiction, but rather as a set of tools you can adapt as you see fit in your own work.

Generating Ideas, Themes, and Data

When you're beginning a work of social fiction, if inspiration has struck, you may already have a topic, theme, story, and/or characters in mind. When that's that case, terrific. You have a starting point. However, if you're interested in developing a project, and you don't yet know what you'd like to focus on, here are some points to consider as you generate ideas.

Like with any other form of research, we typically come to a topic out of a combination of personal interests and experiences, values, and previous research experience. It's also important to consider the significance, value, or worth of writing about a particular topic. This is where your ethical compass comes to bear. To begin, does this topic align with your values system, sense of morality, or political orientation? Is there a social justice imperative to learning more about this topic? Is it important, in relative terms, to write about this topic? Is it timely? Do current events, for instance, make it important to write about this topic at this historical moment? For example, my novel *Film* has undertones of the #MeToo movement. *Film* follows three women who moved to Los Angeles, each to pursue a different creative dream, and the struggles that ensue. Flashbacks are used to show experiences of harassment and assault in each character's past, so readers can see how the experiences at the age of 16 have ripple effects a decade or more later. Primary questions guiding the writing process included: What does the pursuit of happiness look like for women in the context of sexual harassment, assault, and discrimination? How do #MeToo experiences shape women's lives? For another example, authors such as Shalen Lowell, Alexandra C. H. Nowakowski, and J. E. Sumerau have penned social fiction novels centering on nonbinary and transgender characters in an effort to combat current waves of transphobia. Bear in mind that your initial topic or theme may merely be a jumping-off point. Thematic content builds as we write, becoming layered.

As you develop a topic to explore in your writing, consider some of the following questions:

- What is the story you want to tell?
- What are the issues, experiences, themes, and/or micro–macro connections you want to explore?
- What is your objective in writing about this topic or issue?
- What do you hope to evoke in readers?
  o Resonance
  o Empathetic engagement and/or sympathy
  o Raising critical or political consciousness
  o New learning about a particular subject matter or sociohistorical topic
  o Building bridges across differences
  o Unsettling stereotypes and/or disrupting dominant ideologies

Although issues of your potential audience will need to be identified at some point as you select a genre and other critical components to structure your writing, it's never to early to start thinking about who your readers will be. For example, if you want to write a work of fiction that taps into issues raised by Black Lives Matter, in an effort to promote racial justice, who are the relevant stakeholders you hope to reach with your work? How are you positioned relative to this movement? What stories are you qualified to tell? Who might benefit from hearing those stories? Thinking about your audience early on may influence how you shape your topic as well as the choices that follow.

There is also the question of data generation. The data for a social fiction project can be garnered in different ways. There are two primary approaches to data generation (see Figure 3.1): (1) garnering data from traditional research methods and (2) using writing as the generative act.

Sometimes researchers use traditional data collection methods, such as interviews, field research, or document analysis, and then interpret and represent the data using literary writing strategies. For example, interview transcripts may be coded in order to develop specific themes, and the interviewees may be grouped together on the basis of a finite number of experiences and/or traits. Composite characters may then be constructed out of each of those types. While the result will be a fictional

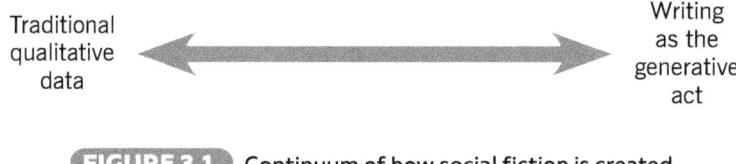

FIGURE 3.1. Continuum of how social fiction is created.

narrative, this process is awfully close to a traditional qualitative interview study. You may also draw from a literature review, using concepts, language, and theories.

In other instances, the writing itself is the generative act, serving as both a method of inquiry *and* form of representation. The writing, as the research act, may be influenced to varying degrees by any number of previous research, teaching, and/or personal experiences as well as concepts and theories from the literature (for example, your writing may follow a feminist or critical race theoretical framework). de Freitas (2003) explains this process as follows:

> The stories are not based on traditional data in the qualitative sense. As a fiction writer, I am always already writing; there is no collecting data before my act of interpretation. There is no temporal lag between event and story. My life experiences as a teacher and a researcher inform my writing, but they are not the "indubitable facts" to which my narrative must correspond. . . . My imagination is immediately engaged in the co-construction of our shared reality. . . . Honour the ways in which my imagination might furnish a form of rigorous research. (p. 1)

In a later work, de Freitas explains that "reflexive writing" is her research methodology (2004, p. 262). Similarly, Dunlop (2001) uses fiction as an act of research. For Dunlop this research practice involves creating an assemblage of "facts" and imagination rendered with literary artifice.

I have used both approaches, although I gravitate toward the latter one in which writing is the generative research act. Writing is my method of inquiry. For novices unsure of what path to follow, it can be useful as you're starting out to mirror a more traditional qualitative research process. As you gain experience and develop more skill as a literary writer, you may wish to take more chances, using the writing process itself as both the method of inquiry and of representation.

Both approaches present unique strengths and challenges that are summarized in Table 3.1.

Building a Structure

The structure of a fictional work gives you its foundation and form. The general structure may be a short story, a novella, or a full-length novel. In short what structure you use depends on how much content you need to create in order to communicate the narrative. Short stories can be quite powerful and can be an excellent way of making an impact in a relatively short read. Novellas allow you to go further with thematic content, characterization, and so forth. Novels are particularly effective for telling a complex story or multiple intersecting or overlapping stories. Novels are also a good choice when deep characterization or plot development is needed to communicate the thematic content or when the story unfolds over a longer period of time.

There are several types of structures to consider when writing a novella or novel. Our understanding of literary structures dates all the way back to Aristotle's book *Poetics*. In the simplest of terms, he maintained that each protagonist has a central conflict that must be faced, and that the action of the dramatic work take place in two acts. Other writers and philosophers have since proposed various structures. Perhaps most famously, Gustav Freytag (1863) developed a five-part dramatic arc that includes exposition, rising action, climax, falling action,

TABLE 3.1. Data from Traditional Research Methods versus Writing as the Generative Act

Data from traditional research methods	Writing as the generative act
Bears similarities to traditional qualitative research (more scientific).	Less like traditional qualitative practice (more artistic).
Provides clear material to develop characters, setting, etc. Requires less imagination.	Requires more imagination to develop characters, setting, etc.
Must maintain fidelity to the data (less freedom).	Allows complete creative freedom.

and resolution. Today most fiction writers adapt modified versions of this format. The primary structures, which are reviewed in detail in Chapters 4–7, include: traditional three-act structures, sequels, open structures, series, and alternative structures (which encompass a broad range of existing possibilities as well as those you may create). Structures aid the organization and pacing of fictional narratives. Structures help you parcel out the story and create flow. Once you've selected your general structure, there are additional elements to consider in order to construct the framework for the narrative: master plots; plot and story line; scenes, narrative, and gaps; and endings, closure, and expectations.

Master Plots

Master plots, sometimes referred to as master narratives, are narratives that are told over and over again in different ways. These stories draw on deeply held values, hopes, and fears (Abbott, 2008). Master plots frequently reappear in the literature within a given culture, and at times, across cultures. Some master plots—the quest story, the story of revenge, for instance—are essentially universal, while others are more culturally specific (Abbott, 2008). The classic Cinderella story is an example of a master plot that reappears in different guises.

Master plots are powerful literary tools because they resonate deeply with readers and therefore carry "enormous emotional capital" (Abbott, 2008, p. 46). Using a master plot allows us to draw on that emotional capital. Sometimes writers unconsciously adapt a master plot. As researchers using fiction, it is worthwhile to consider the possible advantages of tapping into a narrative that readers are likely to find familiar, credible, and resonant. In truth, master plots are so broad that a writer would be hard pressed to write a story that doesn't adapt one. So while we all strive for originality in our fiction, it's also important to be realistic. Most stories have been told many times. Perhaps it's best to ask yourself how you'll tell it differently.

Plot and Story Line

A plot refers to the overall structure of the narrative. Typically the process of plotting involves ordering the major events or scenes of the story and sketching a general outline of the beginning, middle, and end of the narrative. Major "plot points" are typically noted during this process.

For example, a traditional three-act structure includes narrative exposition, an inciting incident or central conflict, and resolution. When you're devising a plot, note what generally happens at these different points of the narrative.

The story line refers to the progression or sequence of events within the plot (Saldaña, 2003). The plot is a general A to B to C. The story line fills in the details of how you get from A to B and so on. Story lining can be an involved process. Whereas you may have a clear sense of the overall plot—what generally transpires in the beginning, middle, and end of the narrative, including the narrative arc—how you get from A to B to C is much more complicated. Some writers draft a detailed story line at the outset. This is a strategy that works for many; however, other writers prefer to work with a general plot structure and fill in the story line as they write. Similarly, some writers have a general plot structure and parts of the story line sketched and fill in the rest throughout the writing process. Everyone's approach to writing is different and even differs with each project, and you should develop a process that works for you. If you do choose to write a detailed story line in advance, it's important to remain flexible and open to the process of discovery. Sometimes a character will reveal something you hadn't anticipated and the story will take a turn, altering a scene or creating a domino effect, whereby everything that follows must shift from your original plan. This is part of the fun of writing fiction. Insights develop as you write. Allow yourself the freedom to follow new learning.

Scenes, Narrative, and Gaps

There are two basic methods used in writing fiction: scenes and narrative. Fictional writing typically draws on both approaches, although that's not always the case.

Scenes are a dramatic way of writing—by showing what is happening as if the action were unfolding before the reader's eyes. Well-written scenes offer a heightened sense of realism and appear like slices of reality or episodes (Caulley, 2008, drawing on Gutkind, 1997). When you are writing in a scenic or dramatic fashion you "write about one continuous action in essentially one place by essentially the same people" (Cheney, 2001, p. 27). Cheney (2001) writes:

> As fiction writers know, scenes give vitality, movement, action—life—to the story. Scenes show people doing things, saying things, moving

right along in light of ongoing stream. Even when writing about the past, writers may play scenes in the present tense, giving the reader the feeling of being eyewitness to the action. (p. 11)

Scenes are about *showing*. On a practical note, scenic writing may involve the use of active verbs (Caulley, 2008).

Narrative writing, on the other hand, is a means of summarizing or offering readers information beyond what is transpiring in specific scenes. Narrative writing is less about showing and more about *telling* (Caulley, 2008). It can be helpful in communicating information that happened outside of the scenes and/or providing commentary on characters and/or situations. This kind of writing typically involves the use of passive verbs. The narrator's voice emerges when employing third-person narration. For example, narrators may explain background information about characters in order to contextualize or comment on situations that have occurred in the past or present. Let's look at an example. The excerpts shown in Table 3.2 are from Chapter 13 of my novel *Shooting Stars*, a love story.

TABLE 3.2. Scenic versus Narrative Writing

Scenic writing	Narrative writing
She answered his FaceTime call, seated in the library stacks, her glasses askew. She whispered, "Hey, baby. They don't allow cell phone use. You're going to get me in trouble." "I just wanted to see your pretty face," he said quietly. She smiled. "How's it going?" he asked. "I just read the most fascinating study about how our brains process literature. I'll tell you about it tonight, but for now, I really need to go. I have a lot to get through and the reference librarian is giving me dirty looks." "Okay, sweetheart. I'll see you tonight. How about I pick up takeout?" "Sounds great. Love you." "I love you too," he said.	Days passed, each one easier than the last. Tess was immersed in her book project, Jack was back to feeling fully invested at work, they saw their friends every Friday night, and each day they laughed and loved more. They were happy. On the Wednesday exactly six weeks from the day Jack found Tess hiding in the closet, something changed.

As you can see, the scenic style excerpt occurs in real time as unfolding action. The narrative style excerpt is written from the narrator's perspective and provides a summary. The narrative excerpt I selected also provides an ideal opportunity to review the issue of gaps in fictional narratives.

Fictional narratives by nature are always incomplete. Stories have gaps that readers inevitably fill in (Abbott, 2008; Barone & Eisner, 2012; Iser, 1980). Goldman writes that we interpret a fictional work as we read and "our imaginations fill out the fictional worlds beyond what is explicitly stated" (2013, p. 6). Typically fictional narratives combine scenes and narrative that may occur over some expanse of time, and therefore there are temporal gaps (gaps between scenes). For example, there's a scene that takes place in the evening. The next scene begins the next morning. There is a temporal lag. Sometimes the gaps are much larger. For example, a scene occurs one day. The next scene occurs days, weeks, or months later. Even in cases in which the entire fictional narrative occurs in one dramatic scene (a continuous unfolding action), what happened before and after the scene is still left up to the reader's imagination. Based on what information the author provides about a character, for example, readers will develop their own backstory beyond the words on the page. Like everything else in fiction, gaps are intentional and should be constructed purposefully. Gaps in the narrative allow readers to use their imaginations, and thereby they allow for a multiplicity of meanings to emerge in spaces of ambiguity (Barone & Eisner, 2012, drawing on Iser, 1980). Decide when you want readers to fill in the blanks.

On the subject of gaps, I'll share one of my favorite reader comments to illustrate that the experience of reading fiction involves interpretation. Years ago, I virtually joined an undergraduate class that had read one of my novels. During my remarks, I mentioned that I intentionally did not describe what the protagonist looks like, other than noting she has brown hair—which is just about as generic as you can get. The character was obsessed with the belief that she was not beautiful, so I intentionally didn't describe her, so that readers could imagine her in their own way, even seeing themselves in her. A student protested and said I had described her. We went back and forth, as he insisted he knew exactly what she looked like. I asked him to find a place in the book where I described her appearance. He couldn't. He said, "I was sure you wrote it." I responded, "I didn't. You wrote it. You wrote in your imagination."

Endings, Closure, and Expectations

How do you structure the end of your narrative? The ending is the final impression with which you leave readers. It's their final thought and carries the power to elevate the whole story and leave it lingering in people's minds, or it can be disappointing and forgettable. Because endings have such a big job, it's important to think about what you want to achieve. There are two interrelated issues to consider: expectations and closure.

Readers develop expectations as they read stories. These expectations are based on (1) signs and signals the writer has created and (2) their previous experiences reading stories or even watching television and film. Beginning with the former, there are many different ways that writers create expectations. For example, when the author is working with a familiar genre, readers expect the writing will follow the conventions of that genre. I'm not implying that this needs to be the case, only that those expectations will have been created. Typically in a romance novel readers expect the main characters to fall in love and live happily ever after. Chekhov famously told an aspiring writer "if in the first chapter you say that a gun hung on the wall, in the second or third chapter it must without fail be discharged" (Abbott, 2008, p. 60). The assumption is that by noting there is a gun on the wall the author has set up expectations in the reader and that the author has an obligation to fulfill those expectations. While the former claim may well be true, as readers are accustomed to looking for signs, signals, and foreshadowing, the latter one is open to debate. Expectations do not necessarily need to be fulfilled. In fact, sometimes it is beneficial to violate readers' expectations (Abbott, 2008). A surprise ending may illuminate something we wish to highlight, may point to the constructed nature of the genre or master plot we are drawing on, and/or may require readers to reflexively revisit previously held assumptions, which may in fact be our goal. This brings us to the issue of closure.

Closure refers to "resolution of the story's central conflict" (Abbott, 2008, p. 57). Readers anticipate the ending of the story and will often judge whether an ending is good based on how well it satisfies their expectations. In short readers don't want to be disappointed. Master plots, for example, typically end in anticipated ways, providing closure and familiarity. As an author you will need to decide whether or not to provide closure in a way that fulfills readers' expectations. It's important to be mindful of readers and what their experience of the story may be, but by the same token, we have to stay true to our visions. Sometimes we have good reason for ending a narrative differently than what may be expected. Figuring out how to end a narrative is a balancing act between understanding the expectations readers are likely to develop and deciding when it is appropriate to fulfill them and when it is appropriate to violate them. For instance, in my novel *Low-Fat Love*, some readers thought the protagonist was going to end up with another male character. I violated genre norms when she didn't end up in a romantic relationship with anyone. I did so because in that book it was important that the character learn to have a better relationship with herself. It wasn't about whether or not she had a love interest. I was also attempting to subvert the dominant narrative in pop culture that suggests romantic relationships are the be-all and end-all for women. In short I violated readers' expectations in order to tell the story I thought needed to be told. Some readers loved it. I'm sure others didn't. That's okay.

Style

While structure gives form to literary writing, there are a range of stylistic choices that give fiction its feeling or gestalt. What kind of story are you writing? What's the style of the writing? What feeling do you want to impart? What's the tone or mood? How are you telling the story? There are specific elements that respond to these questions and allow writers to develop a fictional style.

Genres

A genre is a "recurrent literary form" (Abbott, 2008, p. 49). Genres are thematically driven. Popular examples include but are not limited to romance, mystery/suspense, thriller, adventure, speculative fiction, science fiction, inspirational, fantasy, horror, historical fiction, young adult, LGBTQIA, and women's fiction or chick lit. Each genre comes with its own set of conventions, so it's important to familiarize yourself with writing in that genre. This does not mean that you need to follow all the traditional conventions; however, it's vital to be aware of them so that you know when you are meeting or violating readers' expectations. Those decisions should be thoughtful and intentional.

When selecting a genre, first consider the thematic content you wish to cover—your purpose—and allow the content to guide you toward appropriate genres. Second, consider your intended audience. Who do you hope reads the piece? Different genres tend to appeal to different primary audiences. You want to pick a genre your readers will enjoy and find resonant. Finally, remember that master plots are typically linked to particular genres (Abbott, 2008). The decision to use a master plot may go hand in hand with your choice of genre. For example, if you're drawing on the classic Cinderella story master plot, that choice may direct you to either the romance or women's fiction genre.

> If you're a fan of the genre in which you're writing, then you're already familiar with its conventions. If you'd like to write in a genre with which you aren't terribly familiar, read as much as you can in that genre. Wide reading will help you learn its conventions. Once you have a thorough understanding of how a genre typically works, you can make conscious choices about when to follow norms and when to defy them.

Themes and Motifs

A theme is a recurrent idea and a motif is a recurrent subject, idea, or theme. Themes and motifs give fiction layers of meaning. This idea is likely already familiar to you if you've conducted qualitative research. Qualitative researchers are accustomed to thinking and writing thematically. Typically data are coded so that themes may emerge, which then become the focal point of the interpretive and writing processes. When writing social fiction, we often wish to explore and convey thematic content. To do so, we weave themes and motifs into the narrative. They become part of the subtext underscoring the narrative and the substantive content within it. While you may develop themes and motifs from the outset, they will also unfold through the writing process itself. There will be opportunities to reify or layer themes. This is part of the fun of it. For example, in *Celestial Bodies: The Tess Lee and Jack Miller Novels* (Leavy, 2022), darkness and light are twin themes. They are built into the narrative of each novel in numerous ways—through direct discussion of this topic, the repeated use of certain words, the creation of mood or atmosphere, the expression of feelings—and it's further symbolized in material items from clothing to black-and-white photography.

Style and Tone

Every author leaves his, her, or their fingerprint on their writing. An author's style is their unique way of writing—their unique voice. When we gravitate toward certain authors it's not only because the genre they write in may appeal to us, but there's something about their writing in particular that we enjoy—something unique that makes their writing different from someone else's. Fiction relies heavily on writers using their imaginations in conjunction with a range of literary tools that can be made their own. Therefore, styles vary widely. Some elements that contribute to an author's style include sentence structure, attention to the dramatic effects of language (e.g., the use of short statements; of long, flowery statements; or of emotionally weighted language), attention to the lyrical nature of language, the use of humor, the balance between scenic and narrative writing, point of view, narrator voice, and how interior monologue and dialogue are used. The more you write fiction, the more you'll develop your own style based on the skills you learn, your personality, and your preferences.

As you develop your style, I suggest beginning from an authentic place. I like to use humor in my novels, largely as a means of adding lightness to heavier subjects. As a professor, I always incorporated humor into my lectures. When I began writing my first novel, I peppered the narrator's voice with my own brand of humor. This came naturally to me. Sometimes I would find myself laughing as I wrote. Experience has shown me that if you react to your writing—whether it be with laughter or tears—others are likely to do so as well. The more experience I gained as a fiction writer, the better able I've been to weave humor into my writing through characters' voices and not only through narration, and I've learned how to improve my style in other ways too.

> When you've read fiction in the past, it's likely been a leisure time activity. There may be certain authors to whom you gravitate because you like their style, but you've probably approached their writing primarily as a reader. Now it's time to *study* their work. Read fiction by your favorite authors and focus specifically on aspects of their writing that engage you and from which you derive satisfaction. Your goal is not to mimic these authors, but to draw inspiration from them to help you focus on the stylistic aspects that appeal to you.

As you develop your writing style for a particular project, consider the tone of the story. Everything from sentence structure to uses of language to uses of humor and the like will affect the tone of the narrative. Stylistic choices therefore should be made with tone in mind. Consider the following questions:

- What feeling-world do you want to create?
- What emotional response do you hope to prompt in readers? For example, is the story meant to be uplifting, hopeful, tragic, humorous, or suspenseful?
- What is the emotional arc or journey you want to take readers on?

Characterization

Fiction is character driven. Characters are the people who populate your story-world. At the end of the day, readers will forgive many things, but only if they are invested in the characters. This doesn't always mean that they like the characters per se, but they want to go along with them on their journey. Most characters are neither wholly "good" or "bad." Like real people, characters have flaws, challenges, and struggles that make them believable and relatable. To me, the most important part of writing fiction is creating authentic characters—whether they happen to be ordinary, extraordinary, or even aspirational people, they need to be written truthfully and authentically. When writing social fiction, it's also vital to portray people sensitively, compassionately, and responsibly, regardless of whether your characters are based on research participants or wholly imaginative. Avoid or challenge stereotypes. Strive to achieve multidimensionality. Make these fictional folks seem *real*. Treat them with care.

How do you develop characters? This depends on how you've generated data for the project. When using data garnered from traditional research methods (e.g., interviews or field research), characters may be based on research participants. In these instances, there are two primary issues to consider. First as in any research practice there is an ethical obligation to protect the participants' identities. Be careful what details you reveal. Generally speaking you want to create characters that extend beyond any specific participant. Second you need to decide how many participants to transform into characters. For example, will you create composites based on aggregates of data, or will some participants' stories and experiences be highlighted? How many characters are needed to tell the story? When writing is the entire research act, and the characters are purely fictional, you may draw on cumulative research, teaching, and personal experiences. Regardless of how you develop characters, think about what kinds of people are being portrayed and the function of each character in the overall narrative.

If you're new to writing fiction, I suggest creating a robust character profile for each character in your story. This process will help you develop your characters. Here are some items you can include:

- *Physical description.* The physical description may include status characteristics (e.g., gender, race, ethnicity) age, type of clothing, facial features, and perceived attractiveness. Also consider the point of view from which we learn about the character's physicality. For example, are readers introduced to what the character thinks of his, her, or their own appearance, do we see what a character looks like through the eyes of other characters, or do we learn what a character looks like through descriptions by the narrator?

- *Activities.* How does the character spend his, her, or their time? What are they shown doing? How do they feel about these activities? Consider education, employment, and hobbies.

- *Personality.* What is this character like? For example, is the character funny, sarcastic, shy, loud, or boisterous? What are the character's core values, morals, and ethical guidelines? What motivates this character? What makes the character tick? How does the character make others feel? What kinds of relationships do they have?

- *Name.* Names can carry symbolic meanings. For example, character names may denote age, nationality, and religious background. Names can also be used to make characters more distinct or to give them a common "every person" quality. You may also consider whether or not the character will be referred to by one or more nicknames and what those nicknames signify about the character and/or their relationship to other characters. Sometimes when a character has a nickname or term of endearment that is only used by one other character, it's a way of quickly signifying who is speaking during dialogue-based scenes. This is a writerly trick some authors use. For instance, romantic partners may refer to each other as sweetheart, baby, honey, sugar, darling, love, or some such term that always makes it clear who is speaking. For another example, in *Celestial Bodies: The Tess Lee and Jack Miller Novels* (Leavy, 2022), Tess's best friend Omar calls her Butterfly. There is a reason he does so, linked to the story, which is revealed in the first book, *Shooting Stars*. However, it was also a strategy I employed to always make it clear when Omar was speaking to or about Tess.

Beyond the specifics outlined, when developing a character, keep an eye on the big picture. You want to capture the essence of who this person is and find ways to communicate that essence to an audience. Consider the following questions:

- Who are they at their core?
- What is their central motivation?
- What is their central fear?
- What do they have in common with other characters?
- What makes them unique?
- What are their strengths?
- What are their weaknesses?

Character Types

There are recurring kinds of characters referred to as "types." Character types are often linked to master plots, so if you are working within a master plot to structure your narrative, you may work with a character type as well. For example, a battered wife is a character type, and her story (which centers on a cycle of abuse) is a master plot (Abbott, 2008, p. 49). Just as with master plots, character types may carry emotional and symbolic weight for readers, making them potentially useful tools. Readers' expectations are once again an issue. Readers may expect certain kinds of behaviors or personality traits from common character types, so you'll need to decide when to fulfill and when to disrupt those expectations. In truth, there's a balancing act that occurs when using a recognizable type of character. Although you want to capitalize on the resonance they may already have with readers, you don't want to create a flat or surface-level portrayal. When using a character type, be careful to avoid stereotypes or superficiality. Well-written characters have multidimensionality, specificity, and their own voice.

Dialogue, Interaction, and Interiority

Nothing brings a character to life more than dialogue. Through hearing their voices, seeing how they interact with others, and listening to their streams of consciousness and/or private reactions to people or situations, readers learn who characters truly are. It is not surprising that many writers find writing dialogue the most joyous, and in some cases the most challenging part of their work. There are two main techniques for incorporating dialogue into a fictional work: dialogue with others (via interaction) and internal dialogue.

Fictional narratives often feature "captured conversations," which enhance characterization and serve as snippets of the way people communicate daily (Caulley, 2008, p. 435). Writing dialogue between characters illuminates who individual characters are and how they relate to one another. Realistic dialogue—that which rings true—is an important feature in most fiction. It is a critical tool for both character development and moving the plot forward. Here are some points to consider when writing dialogue:

- The way that a character uses language. This includes the use of formal, informal, and slang language, culturally specific expressions, and so forth. A character's particular style of talking can also shed light on the way he, she, or they react to or feel about particular people or situations.
- The relationships between characters. Through dialogue authors denote familiarity between characters, the comfort level of the characters with one another, the closeness or distance between characters, and many other aspects of their relationships.
- The tenor of conversations. The tone, feeling, or mood of conversations and/or interactions is also communicated through dialogue.
- Additional features of dialogue. It is important to consider the pace of a conversation, pauses, audible signals other than language (e.g., sighs, huffs, snorts, groans, or exaggerated words), gestures (e.g., side-eye, rolling eyes, smirking, or hand waving), expressions, and the context in which the dialogue is unfolding (e.g., if there is a conversation between characters sitting in a restaurant, consider how the waiter approaching the table might impact the conversation).

Dialogue literally and figuratively gives voice to your characters. Dialogue must ring true. This is a critical component of creating compelling characters and a believable story-world. Well-written dialogue engages readers and moves the story forward.

In addition to including dialogue between characters, fiction writers also have the ability to represent interiority—what a character is thinking and feeling, which can be understood as the character's stream of consciousness. The ability to reveal internal dialogue and represent a character's interiority is perhaps the greatest distinction between fiction and other writing forms. Representing interiority allows writers to make visible what is otherwise hidden (Caulley, 2008). In the context of social fiction, you may consider using internal dialogue for any of the following purposes:

- Exploring sociopsychological processes (by giving readers access to what a character thinks and feels about himself, herself, or themselves; in response to interactions with others; and in response to particular events, situations, or circumstances).
- Creating empathetic engagement (getting to know, care for, and sympathize or empathize with characters).
- Establishing micro–macro connections (illustrating how larger social, political, economic, cultural, or historical forces are interpreted by characters and/or how they impact characters).

Internal dialogue can be incorporated into the narrative in different ways (and illustrations are given in later chapters). For example, during a dialogue with others we may also have access to what a character is privately thinking. In these instances, we are learning not only about the individual character, but also about the relationships between characters. Internal dialogue can also be used when characters are by themselves. In these instances, characters may be engaged in an activity (such as exercising), they may be consuming art or media (such as reading a book or watching television), or they may be engaged in a passive activity (such as sitting on a train or lying in bed).

Literary Tools

Fiction is a craft. Good writing matters. I don't say this to intimidate you, only to encourage you to learn to play with the tools of your craft. Yes, I said "play." Try things out, experiment, practice. John Van Maanen reminded ethnographers to adhere to literary standards in their impressionist writing in order to keep readers interested. He encouraged researchers to use "unusual phrasings, fresh allusions, rich language, cognitive and emotional stimulation, puns and quick jolts to the imagination" (2011, p. 106). The same advice applies to authors of social fiction.

Just as plumbers, doctors, scientists, and painters all have tools that allow them to do their work, so too fiction writers have literary tools. Learning how and when to use them is an important part of developing your skills and signature style. We write fiction because it allows us to express what is otherwise inexpressible. The writing may be beautiful, rich, layered, emotional, jolting, or transporting. Literary tools allow us to achieve these ends.

Language

Ultimately the only tool that writers really have available is language. Whether writing dialogue, describing places, or reaching a narrative arc, language is the medium with which we communicate. Writing fiction requires attention to craft and specifically to language. This is a practice that demands time, discipline, patience, and artistry. There are no shortcuts. de Freitas writes, "In my own fiction writing, I plunder my experiences, my language, and my very being, to achieve an exactness in my sentences and paragraphs, grooming them over and over until they match my intentions and my sense of potential impact. Nothing is sloppy in fiction. . . . Composing fiction is a rigorous act" (2004, pp. 269–270). When writing fiction, one must constantly go back to revise, tweak, and rework the language. Of course language imparts meaning, but it does so much more. Consider how words sound, alliteration, the length of words, and how words function when strung together.

Like many novelists, including Stephen King, I'm a believer in writing first drafts on your own. Hear only the voice in your own head. Get lost in the story-world. Translate what you see in your mind's eye. Write as much as you can, knowing you can edit later. Once you've completed a full draft, it's time to engage in cycles of revisions and seeking feedback. Be ruthless when you revise. Red pen every unnecessary word. Be specific with your language. Pay attention to sentence structures, aiming to vary not just what you say, but *how* you say it. Look for and weed out repetition. Use repetition purposefully. Reorganize dialogue and scenes, playing with what you have until you're satisfied. Look for spaces to elaborate and spaces to pare down.

It's also important to seek feedback from peers and mentors. Join or create a writing group or find a writing buddy with whom to share your work. Writing groups and buddies work well when there is an atmosphere of noncompetition and everyone is committed to helping one another best achieve their vision. Sometimes it takes a while to find the right fit, much like finding a romantic partner or therapist. Try to set expectations from the beginning. Professional copy editors are also essential. The best copy editors do more than fix grammar and the like—they point out writing choices that are or are not working well, they make note of tonal issues, and they offer alternatives to trouble spots. When you're sharing your work with those you trust, take in their feedback with gratitude, consider it carefully, stew on it, and try out their suggestions. In the end, you'll need to sort through the feedback you get, to accept those suggestions you find helpful, and to let go of others. Even though feedback is important, you don't want to get mired down with too many different ideas either. Like so much in writing fiction, it's a balancing act of weighing the perspectives others offer as well as your own vision. In the end, the writing should sound like you, the author. Feedback should be used to help you achieve that end, not to derail you.

> Read your work out loud. Taking this step will help you hear what you've written differently than you do when reading in your head, and is enormously helpful during the process of revising. It's also useful for hearing if dialogue rings true—if it sounds the way people actually speak.

Description, Detail, and Specificity

Rich descriptions of places, people, and situations help to draw readers into the narrative. As readers enter into the social world represented in the story, they want to see, hear, and smell what the characters in that space are experiencing. In this regard, the robust descriptions that often characterize fictional writing bear a striking similarity to the "thick descriptions" found in the best ethnographic writing (Geertz, 1973). The way a room looks—in terms of size, color, lightness and darkness, its mood, smell, the objects it contains, how a character feels in that space— may be important. Physical descriptions do more than denote what a person or place looks like; they help create the atmosphere and mood.

During the process of building descriptions, incorporate concrete details. Realistic details "conjure emotions and images in the reader" (Caulley, 2008, p. 447). When writing about qualitative inquiry, Johnny Saldaña urges researchers to document "rich, telling details about a participant or field site that capture an essence or quality" (2018, p. 28). Change *participant* to *character* and *field site* to *setting* and the same holds true for social fiction. Details matter. The use of details accomplishes several things in social fiction. First, these details create mood or atmosphere and help develop the tone of the narrative. Second, incorporating realistic details helps us achieve verisimilitude. Achieving authenticity paves the way for creating resonance and prompting reader engagement. Finally, as researchers we are incorporating empirical data and/or details into our stories, whether these empirical details come from traditional data generation or our cumulative experiences that shape the writing process. Selecting and combining this empirical data, as Iser (1997) suggested, is an integral part of the fictionalizing process. The selection and combination of realistic details or data are central strategies for weaving themes or motifs into a narrative.

Writing fiction well requires specificity. Use language clearly and crisply to achieve your intention. Every word conveys meaning. Is the sky blue, or cobalt, or starry? Is the water 300 degrees or scalding? Is she sad, melancholy, depressed, or defeated? Is he heartbroken, gutted, or shattered? Be specific.

Foreshadowing and Flashbacks

Foreshadowing is a way for writers to hint at what is coming up later in the narrative. While it is used in the construction of a plot and could have been discussed earlier, because it is a literary device, I've chosen to briefly discuss it here. Foreshadowing is often understood to create suspense, build anticipation, and foster dramatic tension. While it can be used in that way, it is by no means the only way. Sometimes foreshadowing is simply used as signposting, a method of dropping clues or advance warnings, often subtly, about events to come. I think of it like leaving a trail of breadcrumbs for readers. These hints may or may not be noticed as they occur, but ultimately help to construct a cohesive narrative that all comes together. In the case of a series or serial, foreshadowing can even be used at the end of a novel to signal what will happen in the next one. For example, in my novel *Constellations*, toward the end of the book, Tess, the protagonist, tells her husband Jack, "Nothing could ever come between us." Indeed, in *Supernova*, the next book in the series, something happens that threatens to pull them apart.

Flashbacks are a common device for providing a backstory. Flashbacks take you to something that happened earlier in a character's life.

This device is used to help you learn more about characters, how they've become who they are now or how they've arrived at their present circumstances, and to contextualize and shed light on their current situation. In Chapter 5 multiple examples of flashbacks are presented. In Chapter 6 I present storytelling as an alternative to flashbacks, in which a backstory may be provided without sacrificing the continuity of the unfolding action.

Metaphors, Similes, Symbolism, and Juxtaposition

Fiction writers employ a range of devices in order to achieve rhetorical effect. It's not simply about the language we use, but how we arrange that language to convey meaning and express our ideas more powerfully. There are many rhetorical devices available to writers, a few of which I review here.

Creative writing often draws on the power of metaphors and similes. Metaphors are used to create a link or comparison between two ideas. For example, in my novel *Supernova*, I use the concept of supernovas (a stellar explosion that gives birth to new stars) as a metaphor to talk about the relationship between the two protagonists during a crisis point. Similes are used to directly compare two ideas by highlighting their similarity to each other using words such as "like" or "as." Crazy like a fox is a common simile. If you're approaching social fiction from a qualitative research background, draw on that experience. Qualitative researchers are adept at thinking metaphorically and symbolically (Saldaña, 2011). Metaphors and similes can be used to enhance the aesthetic quality of any work of fiction, but there are added benefits for social fiction. They may be used to create micro–macro connections; to challenge, disrupt, or subvert taken-for-granted assumptions; or to create subtext. They "allow writers both to interpret and construct meanings" (Watson, 2016, p. 12).

Fiction writers also often use symbolism to build and impart meaning. Symbolism allows writers to convey meaning in an artistic or poetic, as opposed to a literal, way. For instance, a writer might use shades of blue to denote sadness or depression and instill a melancholic tone, instead of directly describing characters as depressed. For another example, stormy weather or unwieldy landscapes might be used as symbolism for troubled relationships. Let's look at a brief example from my own work. The collection *Celestial Bodies: The Tess Lee and Jack Miller Novels* (Leavy, 2022) centers on themes of darkness and light. Symbolism is woven throughout the novels to reify that theme, for example, through black, white, and gray clothing, black-and-white photographs, black-and-white galas, and references to the sky at different times of day.

The preceding example of darkness and light leads me to a final literary tool: juxtaposition. Juxtaposition involves placing two subjects side by side in order to highlight their differences. It's a commonly used tool for creating contrast. Any two subjects—characters, places, concepts, or objects—may be contrasted. For example, two male characters may appear in one scene—one exhibiting misogyny and another positive masculinity. The stark contrast between the two serves to amplify certain traits in each character, while simultaneously highlighting the differences between the two.

Front and Back Matter

When writing a novel, there are several ways of book-ending the story or packaging it for readers, with front and back matter content. These parts are optional, and your novel may include any number of these parts or none at all.

Prologues and Epilogues

Prologues and epilogues are *parts of the story,* each set in a time before and after the main narrative. A prologue is an opening to a novel that provides context or background information. It may be set anywhere from years to merely a day before the main narrative begins. An epilogue is an ending to a novel that occurs after the main narrative has concluded, whether that be the next day or years later. An epilogue provides closure or "where are they now" information not contained in the main text. For example, my novel *The Location Shoot* (Leavy, in press) opens with a prologue written as an entertainment news report. It is used to introduce the characters and set up the action of the novel. The epilogue, also in the form of an entertainment news report, follows up months later on what happened to the characters after the novel's final scene. For another example, all the novels in *Celestial Bodies: The Tess Lee and Jack Miller Novels* (Leavy, 2022) include an epilogue, anywhere from a day to a year after the novel ends. The epilogue shows where the characters are now, illustrating the ways in which what they've learned over the course of the story has affected their lives, and sums up the themes from the book.

Forewords, Prefaces, and Afterwords

Forewords, prefaces, and afterwords are front and back content that are *not* a part of the novel itself, but are written in the author's or a guest author's voice. A foreword is a short introduction to a novel that is written by someone other than the author. A preface is a short introduction to a novel that is written by the author. While in fiction it's far more common to have a foreword than a preface, in the case of social fiction, some authors like the opportunity to talk about their intent in writing the novel and/or the research or other experiences that informed it. If a book includes both a foreword and preface, the foreword appears first. An afterword is placed at the end of the novel and is a short discussion of the book that may include why or how it was written. An afterword may be written by the author or someone else. In the case of social fiction, it is another opportunity for an author to talk about their intention and/or process.

Again, all these front and back matter elements are optional and should be used in accordance with your specific goals.

Titles

You've penned a work of fiction. What do you call it? Titles are incredibly important and they're also very personal. The title signals to potential readers what the work of fiction is about. It's also something that you as an author should feel good about—it should mean something to you and as closely as possible "match" what you feel is most important about the work. A title might be direct or might be something readers will not fully understand until they've read the entire work. Sometimes we know the title before we start writing. And sometimes, the title doesn't reveal itself until the end. There's no one way to approach titling your work, and I myself have used different strategies. For example, I've spent months contemplating the concept the book ultimately conveys, and that process led me to the title *Low-Fat Love* for my debut novel. In some cases, I've known the title from the start, as for my novel *Shooting Stars,* in which the title means something significant and different from what readers may expect and the meaning is not revealed until the last chapter. When you're writing a sequel or serial, one title might lead to another, as in the Tess Lee and Jack Miller serial I wrote; each novel has a celestial-themed title, and in each case the title relates directly to the main lesson learned in the book. When you're trying to develop a title, I suggest the following:

- As you write, keep a running list of key words and phrases that stand out to you in your book.
  - Look for synonyms for those words to come up with additional possibilities.
- Note key themes, concepts, or metaphors as possible titles.

Once you have a working title, play around with it. I believe that generally less is more. If you can eliminate extra words, do so.

Conclusion

As I've noted from the outset, there is no cookie-cutter approach to writing social fiction. However, I hope the ideas and strategies reviewed in this chapter are helpful as you develop your own writing practice and style. When it comes to writing, the two pieces of advice I always return to are these: have fun with it and revise, revise, revise.

I would be remiss not to raise the issue of what happens when you publish your fiction: reader response. We never know how an audience will respond to our creative writing. Fiction is a uniquely personal form of writing, and so authors are likely to feel particularly attached to their work and sensitive to audience reaction. This is normal. We love our fiction and feel close to it. We know every detail about it and the characters become a part of our soul and, in a way, our own life story. It's natural to feel protective of them. However, the reality is that fiction is highly subjective and readers may respond in all sorts of ways, from feeling deeply connected to what we've created to outright hating it. The best advice I can give you, which has carried me through the years, is this: develop your own relationship with your writing that isn't dependent on anything external. You can't control readers' responses to your work, so don't try to, and don't get caught up in them. The relationships readers develop with characters and stories is theirs, not yours, and that's how it should be. Realize that praise can be just as damaging to creativity as critique. In both cases, it's an external measure of your work. Again develop your own relationship with your creative writing. This will allow you to continue to write freely and share your work, regardless of the response, which for most authors is always a mixed bag with highs and lows. While you're working on your story, seek feedback in the ways I suggested or whatever ways suit you. Be ruthless in editing your own work—you may need to revise a chapter more than two dozen times to get it "just right" and whittle it down to tightly crafted prose. However, once you've decided the piece is done, let it go. Make peace with it and let it go.

> **SKILL-BUILDING EXERCISE** Using the topic you selected at the end of Chapter 1, create a character (meant to be a protagonist). For example, if your topic is centered on education, your character may be a student, teacher, or administrator. If your topic is centered on health care, your character may be a nurse, doctor, orderly, lab technician, patient, caregiver, or medical researcher. Name the character and develop a robust character profile that includes a physical description, main professional and leisure-time activities, and personality. Describe the character's values, motivations, challenges, and family and friendship network. Consider the people who populate their world.

> **RETHINK YOUR RESEARCH** Select one of your research participants and transform them into a character or select several participants who share similarities and create a composite character. (If you don't have research participants, create a character based on yourself as you relate to the research project.) Name the character and develop a robust character profile that includes a physical description, main professional and leisure-time activities, and personality. Describe the character's values, motivations, challenges, and family and friendship network. Consider the people who populate their world.

4 Traditional Three-Act Structures

> Techniques highlighted in this chapter:
> ✓ Dialogue
> ✓ Internal dialogue/interiority
> ✓ Third-person narration

There are several traditional structures that novelists employ, including five-act, four-act, and three-act structures. The most common one is the three-act structure that divides a story into three acts or parts: the set-up, the confrontation, and the resolution. The first act, the **set-up**, is typically used for **narrative exposition**. The primary characters are introduced, the relationships between the characters are fleshed out, the setting is established, and to varying degrees a backstory is provided. As part one moves along, there is an **inciting incident**, which introduces drama into the narrative, and may occur at the end of part one. At this critical point in the plot, something challenges the protagonist, which ultimately must be confronted. The second act centers on the **confrontation, central conflict, or rising action** in the novel, which typically worsens as this part of the story unfolds. The protagonist often lacks the means to solve the problem off the bat, and so things get worse before they get better. This is the central part of the protagonist's journey, during which they change, grow, and evolve. This transformation is referred to as a **character arc**.

The third and final act offers **resolution or revelation**, as the protagonist completes his, her, or their journey (and supporting characters do as well).

This strategy for organizing a plot builds dramatic tension into the narrative. Events may be going along swimmingly or unremarkably in act one until the conclusion when conflicts begin to arise, ending that part of the book in a way that leaves readers wanting to come back for more. Then, in part two, as conflicts unfold the drama increases correspondingly, reaching a climax and leaving readers to wonder: Will it be a turning point? Will things work out? How will the protagonist fair? Last, in the final part, all questions are answered as the characters reach resolutions.

Low-Fat Love

Low-Fat Love was my debut novel. I began writing it during a sabbatical after reflecting on my professional and personal life. For nearly a decade I had collected interview research about women's lives. For even longer I had taught undergraduate courses on topics that included gender, sexuality, and popular culture. Cumulatively I learned a great deal through my research and my encounters with students, both inside and outside of class, yet I had nowhere to share those insights. There were also personal experiences with past relationships stewing in my mind that needed resolution. So one day I took some of my informal notes or jottings and started penning my first novel—an exploration of women's identity, self-esteem, and relationship struggles.

Low-Fat Love follows a three-act structure. The novel unfolds over three seasons as Prilly Greene and Janice Goldwyn, adversarial editors at a New York City press, experience personal change relating to the men in their lives. Without meaningful female friendships or support systems, these women suffer in isolation within the context of unhealthy relationships. Ultimately each is pushed to confront her own image of herself, exploring her insecurities, the stagnation in her life, her attraction to men who withhold their support, and her reasons for having settled for low-fat love. Prilly, the protagonist, lives in between who she is and who she longs to be. Prilly moved to New York in search of a "big life." Convinced that only beautiful women can truly have their heart's desire, and fearing she is "in the middle" (not beautiful or ugly), she resigns herself to the idea that she'll have to work harder than others for her shot at the life she aspires to. After a chance meeting at a bookstore, she falls for Pete Rice, a sexy and curiously charming aspiring graphic novelist. Suddenly everything she's ever longed for is within her grasp. However, Pete's unconventional, free-spirited views on relationships unsettle Prilly, eventually causing her to unravel over the course of their on-again-off-again love affair. Meanwhile, Janice, a workaholic, feminist-in-name-only editor, overburdens her with busywork and undercuts Prilly's professional identity. Janice's regimented life is set on a new course when her alcoholic father becomes injured in a car accident and she is forced to face her own demons. The stories of additional supporting characters—each of whom struggles with issues of self-esteem, identity, relationships, and loneliness—are woven into the novel.

The following three excerpts are from parts one, two, and three of the book, respectively. They represent the inciting event in part one, the confrontation in part two, and the resolution in part three. Together they are meant to illustrate these primary aspects of a three-act narrative structure. These extracts follow the central relationship between Prilly and Pete, and ultimately the relationship Prilly has with herself as she struggles with her own self-esteem and self-concept in the context of this toxic relationship.

The first excerpt is from Chapter 4, as we're nearing the end of part one. Prilly's boss has informed her that Janice has complained about her at work, after which she raced out of the office, hurrying to meet Pete as she did each night, stopping to freshen her makeup in a Starbuck's restroom. Insecure that Pete is too good for her, she relentlessly tries to be interesting, to accommodate his schedule, and to look her best at all times, racing around the city with a full makeup bag. I selected this extract because it is the inciting incident that gives way to the forthcoming central conflict. The second excerpt is from Chapter 7 in part two. In an earlier chapter set on Halloween, Pete and Prilly bumped into his ex-girlfriend Clyde at a party, leading the couple to have their first huge blowout argument. Six weeks later, it comes to a head. The final excerpt is taken from the last chapter in part three. After more push and pull in their relationship, Prilly thought she had let Pete go. However, when Pete's friend Melville disappears, and is presumed dead, he calls her, and they meet one last time. Prilly was aware that there were parallels between how Pete treated her and how he treated Melville. Melville had also been insecure and unsure of himself and Pete always spoke to him as if he were beneath him, and yet Melville always returned for more. In this final scene between Pete and Prilly, we get the resolution or revelation.

Low-Fat Love, Excerpt from Chapter 4

"She's just so two-faced," Prilly said as she maneuvered some lo mein into her mouth.

"Here, let me show you. You're not holding them right," Pete said as he illustrated how to properly place one's fingers on chopsticks.

Embarrassed, Prilly tried to copy him, but moments later resorted back to her own way of holding them.

"Well, is there any truth to it? Have you been pulling your weight?" Pete matter-of-factly asked as he knocked a container of spicy pea pods over onto the old towel that lay across the bed as a makeshift tablecloth.

Unable to control her frustration at what felt like the second betrayal of the day, Prilly snapped back, "She's just a bitch. Don't you get it? I'm doing *most* of the work, not just a little, but most of it. And I never wanted to do this in the first place—she bullied me into it. What the hell is that to say something to my boss when she hasn't said a word to me? She's obviously up to something."

"Well then, you've got to confront her. Take the venom out of it." Before Pete could continue his phone rang. He leaned over and grabbed it off the floor. "Hello?" He turned his back and lowered his voice. "Hey, this isn't a great time. I'm eating with a friend.... Where? What's the address? ... I'll try to make an appearance, but no promises.... Yeah. Okay, bye."

Friend??? Prilly thought. *Am I just a friend?* she wondered, as the speed of her animosity built like a runaway car on a rollercoaster straight out of a childhood nightmare.

"Who was that?" she asked most curiously.

"A friend of mine, Clyde. She's having some issues, just broke up with some guy, blah blah blah. She wants to see me. She's going to a small gothic club downtown in a bit. She was hoping I'd make an appearance."

"Oh. Well, I thought we were gonna stay in tonight. I'm tired and upset. I don't really feel like going to a club."

"How about this: why don't you stay here and relax, maybe read or go to sleep, and I'll slip out for a couple of hours?"

Prilly didn't know what to say. *I can't believe that he would leave me here alone. And who is this woman that he wants to see more than he wants to be with me? A woman to whom I am just "a friend?"* She felt like bursting into tears but refused to show him how upset she was, so she coldly said, "Well, I guess, if that's what you want to do, I can just go home."

"No, no, stay here. Stay, relax, listen to music, eat this food, and I'll be back in a couple of hours."

Pete jumped up and walked to the bathroom, bringing the container of lo mein with him. Prilly just sat there. She heard the shower turn on. She heard it turn off. She heard the sink faucet turn on, then off. She heard him open the bathroom door. She mostly heard the angry voice in her head, a high-pitched voice that wouldn't shut up. She just sat there, silently fuming. All she wanted all day was to be with Pete, and now he was ditching her for some other woman. He came into the room and casually said, "Hey girl," and smiled, as if totally unaware of the angst he was causing her. He put the nearly empty Chinese food container down on the bed and said, "That's delicious. I couldn't stop myself," and laughed. As he bent over, she could smell his newly spritzed cologne. She wanted desperately to remain silent, to stay cool. She had been telling herself over and over and over again during his twenty-five minutes in the bathroom that she needed to play it cool. But after that whiff of his cologne, she blurted out, "Who is this friend? Is she an old girlfriend?"

He chuckled. "If you're asking if I've slept with her, yeah, sure, but we're just friends. She's going through a bad time and she wants to talk. I kind of feel like getting out tonight, and you don't. Even if you did, I don't think it would be the best time to introduce you. I broke up with her, and now she just broke up with someone, and you know."

No, I don't know. I don't know why the man I am crazy about, the man I am running all over town to see while utterly exhausted is leaving me to see another woman whom he's slept with, a woman who may still have feelings for him! She could feel rage brewing and feared it would slip from her lips. She held onto it as tightly as she could, worrying that she might induce a stroke.

He leaned down and kissed her on the forehead. As he bent over she heard his black leather pants squeak. They were tight, and with a long black and silver long-sleeved T-shirt over them, he looked sexy. He smelled good, and he looked sexy. She was livid.

* * *

When Pete left with a "See ya, girl," Prilly experienced physical paralysis and mental Tourette's. She couldn't stop wondering what had just happened. In her mind, over and over again, *What just happened?* Then she started to obsess about Clyde, this woman Pete was so eager to see. She knew he had slept with other women of course, and by his unmatched sexual talents she figured there had been many of them, but she didn't want to think about it; she didn't want to know about them. She mostly didn't want him to care about them. *Clyde, Clyde. She's probably really beautiful. She sounds beautiful. She's probably really cool. She probably wouldn't mind if he ran out to see an old girlfriend. She's probably beautiful.* As she sat in his little apartment that now stunk of Chinese food, a smell she couldn't get rid of long after putting away the leftovers and washing the dishes, she felt sick. The longer she waited, the angrier she got. *Who the fuck is he to leave me like this? What kind of fucking man does this? He doesn't care. He doesn't care about how I feel!*

She decided to get ready for bed and then pretend to sleep until he got home. She wanted to look good, assuming they would make love after he apologized and told her how wonderful she was, so she brushed her teeth but slept with her makeup on. She didn't want to really fall asleep, afraid she would have bad breath and messy hair by the time he returned, so she just lay in bed, thinking, spinning, seething. Four and a half hours passed, with each minute experienced like the labored breaths of an old woman on her deathbed. She twice got up to rinse her mouth with Listerine and to powder her nose. She felt pathetic, really pathetic, and she knew she should just get up and leave without a note or phone call, but instead, she lay there counting the seconds. Her thoughts vacillated from Pete to Clyde to Janice and Stuart. Her big life was shrinking.

Shortly after two-thirty, she heard a key in the door. Pete went straight into the bathroom, and ten minutes later, made his way to the bed where Prilly was still pretending to sleep, afraid he could hear her overpowering heartbeats. When he got into bed, she rustled around a bit so he would think he woke her up. He didn't say anything and she could feel his back to her, so eventually she just went to sleep. She woke up at five in a cold sweat, and then fell back asleep.

The next morning Prilly got up, showered and dressed, and made two mugs of coffee with Pete's one-cup coffee maker. There was only a little cream left, and she used most of it in her coffee. *Screw him.* She stood in the kitchen, looking through the cutout wall, trying to read his mind as he slept. *Am I overreacting? Am I being too sensitive? Did it mean anything? Why didn't we make love when he got home?* She couldn't wait for him to wake up and somehow make it better.

After an hour and forty-five minutes of waiting, trying to subtly make just enough noise to wake him without being obvious, he finally woke up, rubbing his eyes and clearing his throat. "Hey. I smell coffee," he said in a low voice.

"Yeah, I made you a cup. You might have to nuke it, it's been sitting for a while."

"K. Thanks," he said as he stood up, wearing the same long-sleeved T-shirt he had left in, now paired with his black boxers. He lifted his arms high into the air and made a loud yawning noise as he stretched upward. "I have to go to the bathroom. I'll be right there."

The next two minutes seemed somehow to be a hundred times longer than all that preceded them. Prilly stood in the kitchen, sipping her cold coffee, not knowing what to do. Pete came in and kissed her on the forehead, grabbed his coffee, and went to the refrigerator for cream. He spilled the last drops into his mug and said, "We're out of cream."

"I know."

He took his mug and walked past her into the bedroom. He propped his pillow against the wall and sat on the bed, legs outstretched, drinking his coffee. Furious, Prilly made a loud sigh and walked into the bedroom with her mug in hand. She sat in the computer chair, and just as Pete started to smile at her, she said, "So, you got home late last night."

"Yeah, sorry. After midnight I figured you were asleep and that it didn't matter, so I stayed a bit longer. Didn't want to call and wake you."

In a sharp tone she responded, "Well, did you have a good time? Is your friend okay?"

"Oh, you know, she's always going through something. She has a tinsel heart, you know. She's like a bird that you want to take care of."

What the fuck is this? Prilly screamed inside her head. *Doesn't he know how upset I am? Can't he see that I'm upset?* The silent anger quickly turned to hurt. *Tinsel heart? Bird? Is everything about her beautiful? It sounds like he loved her. Maybe he still loves her.* Despite all of the thoughts swimming in her mind, she managed to stay silent. It took a lot of effort, but the more special Clyde sounded, the less she wanted to reveal how uneasy she was with all of this.

"The club was cool. You would like it; we should go sometime. It was very small and dark, and the walls were covered with dark purple fabric, like a flowing translucent kind of fabric. The music was wonderful, a terrific DJ. He played lots of trippy stuff like Portishead. I danced all night."

Fighting every inclination she had, she remained quiet, just looking at him and silently screaming, *What the hell is wrong with you?*

"I'm gonna hop in the shower. Starving. You want to go to that diner again, the one with the fabulous waitress?"

"Sure," she said, feeling relieved that they were spending the day together, but also angry and utterly confused.

Pete got up and went to the bathroom to shower.

* * *

An hour later, they were sitting in the diner, waiting for someone to take their order. "I'm ravenous; feel like I could eat a horse," Pete said. *He seems particularly jolly this morning*, Prilly thought.

"Hmm. So you said."

The waitress walked over, and Pete smirked at Prilly; it was not the waitress with the wonderful face. This much younger waitress had a very long, thin face with long, thin features and elfin ears.

She's a bit birdlike, Prilly thought. *Not a pretty bird, but a bird.* She looked at the nametag on her canary-colored uniform: Ruth. *Clyde is probably a beautiful bird*, Prilly imagined.

"I think I'll try an omelet today," Pete said, as if the waitress knew his regular order, or cared. "With mushrooms and cheese, cheddar cheese."

"What kind of toast?"

"Wheat. With marmalade, not jam."

"And for you?"

"Oh, um, I'll have the blueberry pancakes please."

Shit, Prilly thought to herself. *What am I doing? First the lo mein and now pancakes. I'll have to suck in my stomach all day.*

"So what do you want to do today? There's a Shepard Fairey exhibit at the Guggenheim I'm dying to see. Do you know his work?"

"No."

"Oooh, he's wonderful. He's famous for that Obama poster you know, but his other work, his real work, is marvelous. It's all subversive, like the guerrilla art I told you my friends in London were into. There's a marriage between word and image in the work. Very carefully done. Sharp and sardonic. And the Guggenheim, well fuck, that building is an orgasm itself."

"Uh, huh," Prilly said, totally unable to focus on anything he was saying. She then blurted out, "What happened last night? I mean, you totally ditched me and went out with some woman you've slept with before, and then you don't come home until the middle of the night. Do you know how that makes me feel?" As soon as the words came out, she regretted saying them but was desperate to hear his response.

He laughed. He laughed, and then with a close-mouthed smile, he managed to make her feel even more pathetic than she already felt. "It was nothing. A friend called me and she needed me. You could have come but you weren't up for it. You know how I feel about you. What we have is what we have; it has nothing to do with Clyde or with anyone. It shouldn't matter whether I've slept with her or not."

"Well you might not feel that way if it was you."

"If it were the other way around, I wouldn't care. I know what we have, and I wouldn't worry. I wouldn't want to stop you from doing something you wanted to do."

Unsatisfied, Prilly asked, "Were you . . . were you in love with her?"

"Love? I don't even know what love is. Love is just a word people say to each other. I care about her, sure."

Love is just a word people say to each other? He doesn't even know what love is? What the fuck is he saying? How can he say this when he told me that he loved me? He said it first, and he said it twice. How can he be saying this? Prilly wondered. What she actually said aloud was, "I felt like you abandoned me. I was really upset; you knew I had a bad day at work, and we made plans. Then you just left. What's worse, you left to see some woman you had a relationship with. How did you think that would make me feel?"

Ruth brought the food over. Pete thanked her and started eating immediately, sprinkling salt on his omelet with one hand as he ate a forkful of home fries with the other. Prilly just sat there, staring at him.

A few moments later, he put his fork down and said, "Look, I'm sorry if you were upset. Honestly, I didn't think it was a big deal. I thought you were cool with it."

"Okay, I guess we can just drop it," Prilly responded, not quite sure if she had blown it all into something bigger than it was, but certain she didn't want things to escalate further. She cut up her pancakes, drizzled on some syrup, and ate, trying to convince herself she wasn't really as upset as she was.

After a few bites Pete said, "You know, I don't believe in the traditional monogamy thing. I mean, I thought we were cool, that we had an unspoken understanding, but maybe it's best to lay our cards on the table." Unable to take in the oxygen necessary to comprehend this information or formulate a response, Prilly sat silently. Pete continued, "I mean, we're having a wonderful time and it's very special, so there's no reason to label it. What a person has with one person doesn't diminish what they have with someone else. Like with Clyde. What I had with her doesn't take away from how I feel about you. It's totally different."

Too many thoughts, too many thoughts to process, Prilly frantically thought to herself. She took another bite of blueberry pancake in order to buy enough time to steady her voice. "I don't understand. We've spent every day together since we met." Leaning in and lowering her voice, she said, "You told me you loved me."

He again smiled, close-mouthed. "I said what was in my heart in the moment. I always do and it is always true. This you can count on. So who needs false promises when you have that?"

She thought to herself that maybe this Clyde woman, whoever she was, and she did sound wonderful, could see the beauty in what Pete was saying; she probably could, "tinsel heart" and all, but to Prilly, it just felt hurtful, deeply hurtful. She wondered if they had been in the same relationship at all and she felt foolish.

"I still don't understand. Are you saying that you're seeing other people or that you want to? Did something happen with Clyde last night? Is that why you came back so late?"

He offered up another close-mouthed smile. "No, no, nothing happened with Clyde if that's what this is really about, but even if it had, it wouldn't need to change anything we have. Clyde was once a special person in my life, and she is still sort of in my life, but I haven't slept with her since we broke up before I met you. I think she wanted to last night. She was very vulnerable. But truthfully, all I could think about was you at my place, in my bed, waiting for me. I thought it was sweet how you let me go, how you knew it was okay."

Again, too many thoughts; too many thoughts to process at once, Prilly thought, feeling overloaded. He had thrown so much information at her, and she feared none of it was good. She wanted to be cool. She wanted to be the sweet, cool, tinsel-hearted girl who waited in his bed. But she wasn't. So, she responded sharply, "It would matter to me."

"Look, two people can be together forever and be only with each other, but not because of some artificial promise. I don't believe in that. Sure, you can find a thousand men who will give you hollow promises, but that's not me. That's not what I'm giving you. You have to live moment to moment, and the moments string together. And eventually you can string together a lifetime, but not because of promises, just because it is true to your heart, to your soul. You cannot cage a bird, as they say."

Great, more birds, Prilly thought. "It wouldn't be all right with me if you were with someone else. That's not what I want."

He smiled again, letting out the quietest of laughs as if she were too provincial to understand what he was saying or too insecure to deal with it, the latter of which may well have been true.

"Okay, I understand. If anything were to ever happen with someone else, or if I wanted it to, I would tell you. You have my word. I would be honest with you and you could do as you needed to."

"Okay," Prilly softly said, not knowing how to make this dreadful conversation end in a way that would leave them both sitting there, and ideally in a way that would restore the feeling to her numb feet.

"But I don't want to be with anyone else right now. I like being with you," he said, as if he were giving her a gift. Just as she had so many times in earlier years, she felt like Charlie Brown dumping out a Christmas stocking full of coal.

Low-Fat Love, Excerpt from Chapter 7

Over the next six weeks, Prilly started to unravel. She was consumed by jealous impulses. When Pete was in the shower, she glanced at his cell phone. When glances didn't suffice, she scrolled through his emails, texts, and phone logs. Sometimes when his apartment phone rang, she answered it. Knowing that would probably bother him, she never mentioned those calls. To compensate for her fears, she tried to spend as much time as possible with Pete. She tried to be interesting, she tried to be sexy, and mostly she just tried to be there. No longer wanting to run home after work to get an overnight bag and freshen up, she brought a makeup case to work and left two drawers full of clothes at Pete's. She rushed out of the office as quickly as possible and raced to meet him. Every time she caught him chatting up another woman, she found a way to punish him without telling him why.

One Friday night when she arrived at the teahouse, he was sitting and reading something he had written to some woman. Prilly went out of her way to be rude to the woman, who took the hint and left abruptly. Pete smirked and said, "Hey girl, she noticed my drawing and asked what it was, so we ended up having a nice little chat and I read her something. That's all."

Prilly responded, "I don't care." She put on a happy face that night and then went out of her way to be disagreeable for the rest of the weekend. She refused to go to a house party he wanted to pop in on, she told him the art at a gallery they went to was ugly after he said he loved it, and she made enough noise in the mornings to disrupt his sleep without appearing like she was trying to wake him. Worse than anything she was doing to Pete was the mental anguish she was putting herself through. Every time the phone in his apartment rang, she imagined it was Clyde, but on this and this alone, she bit her tongue.

Then one Friday afternoon she got a call at work. "Hello?"

"Hey babe."

"Pete?"

"Yeah, of course."

"Oh, it's just that you've never called me at work before. Is everything okay?"

"Yeah, everything is fine. Listen, I need to ask you to spend the night at your place. I have a situation I need to deal with."

"What's wrong?" she asked solemnly.

"Nothing girl, just got to take care of something. Come over tomorrow night and we'll spend the rest of the weekend together, all right?"

"Okay, sure. I hope nothing is wrong. If you need something, call me."

"Thanks. Bye."

"Bye."

Prilly hung up the phone wondering what was going on. She was filled with questions that all asked the same things: *Is this about me? Is this about us?*

That evening, she returned to her apartment for the first night in weeks. The first thing she noticed was a foul stench coming from her kitchen. She hadn't taken the garbage out in weeks, and something reeked. As she pulled the drawstring bag out of the plastic can, she nearly hurled. She looked at the bottles under her kitchen sink desperate for an odor-eating product. Absent anything like that, she grabbed a bottle of perfume and sprayed some in each room of her small apartment. It didn't help. She sat on her couch trying to decide whether to order Chinese food, but she was too consumed with thoughts of Pete. *What is going on with him? Why didn't he say why he canceled?* She became increasingly agitated. The putrid smell in her apartment was taunting her. *I shouldn't be here. I should be at Pete's.* She thought about going down to the teahouse in his neighborhood to accidentally run into him, if he was there. Knowing it was too transparent, she decided to order some food and curl up on the couch. An hour later she was eating chicken in a spicy brown sauce with chopsticks, right out of the container, while watching a Lifetime movie about a woman who had an affair with her best friend's husband. She drank half a bottle of red wine and passed out in her work clothes.

The next morning she went through the motions of her former morning routine: French roast coffee and her favorite New York website. She wasn't really looking for something to do; she was just passing time until her plans with Pete, whenever that would be. She wasn't particularly eager to spend time with him but she was desperate to find out how he had spent the evening. After a night of panic, she tried to convince herself that it must be something benign and that she was freaking out for nothing. *If he was spending the night with another woman he would have made up some excuse, but he hadn't. It must be nothing.*

After showering and getting ready, she sat on her couch and tried to figure out what to do. She was having a really good hair day, and her outfit was spot-on. She was wearing a long-sleeved, black, sheath-style dress with black tights and new mauve Mary Jane high heels. *I look good and I don't want to sit at home wasting it. I want Pete to see me before the end of the day when I'll undoubtedly be more haggard looking. I'll throw some work in a bag and go to the teahouse near Pete's. Janice has been on my case to mark up the drafts of the first three memoirs, and with any luck, I'll bump into Pete while I still look good.*

An hour later and a block away from the teahouse, her hands began to tingle. This feeling had become familiar so she knew it would soon pass. As she approached the teahouse, Pete was coming out. Just as her adrenaline was pumping hard with wonder about his reaction to seeing her, Clyde emerged. Tremors coursed through her body as Pete turned and saw her. She wanted to turn around and run away, but concerned with saving face, she kept moving forward.

"Prilly, hey, what are you doing in this neck of the woods? You remember my friend Clyde," he said as he touched Clyde's arm.

"I had some work to do and . . . and there's a problem in my apartment, so . . . so I just thought I'd come and get some work done. My apartment reeks. It's unbearable and I need to work. I didn't think I'd see you."

"I was just going to walk Clyde to the subway, but if you wait I'll come back after," Pete said as if nothing was wrong.

"Pete was nice enough to help me out with something last night. I thought the least I could do was take him for a coffee," Clyde interjected, gently brushing her long bangs from her eye.

Unable to stop thinking about Clyde's beauty, Prilly's tremors morphed into full-on waves of rage. Clearly sensing she was upset, Pete said, "Yeah, I'll tell you about it in a bit, okay? Wait for me."

Unable to control herself she blurted out, "No, no I don't think so. I'm not going to wait," and she turned around and walked away so quickly that she twice tripped on her own feet.

Pete hollered after her. "Hang on there," but Prilly just threw one of her arms up in disgust and kept walking.

When she got home, she went straight into her bedroom where she lay on the bed, too worked up to fall asleep. A few hours later Pete called. "Hello," he said tersely.

She screamed, *"Fuck you"* at the top of her lungs and hung up. She waited for him to call back but he didn't. Prilly knew it was over.

Low-Fat Love, Excerpt from Chapter 18

Prilly was just getting home from work when she heard her phone ringing. She let the machine get it but stopped in her tracks at the sound of Pete's voice. She knew she had the willpower to resist the urge to pick up the phone. If she did it once, she could do it again. But when Pete said that something really awful had happened to Melville and that he needed to speak with her, she gave in and picked up the phone. He begged her to come to his apartment. When she refused, he told her he thought Melville was dead and that he needed her. "Please, please Prill, please come over." She agreed. She changed into tight, dark blue jeans and a flowing, gray baby-doll top, fixed her makeup, and took a cab to his apartment. She arrived an hour after he had called.

She was excited, nervous, and unsure of what she was doing. Her hands trembled as she rang the buzzer. As she approached his apartment, the scene of so many heartbreaking and exhilarating moments, he opened the door, gave her a closed-mouthed smile, and said, "Come on in," in his sexiest voice. She sat on the chair by his desk and watched him open a bottle of wine in the kitchen.

"I think I remember you liked Chianti, right?" he asked.

"Actually, I like Cabernet," Prilly said.

"Oh, that's right," he said blushing. "Well this is fabulous. You'll love it. I'm sure it's better than what you normally have."

"Pete, what's going on? I didn't come for a social call. You said Melville might be dead. Were you exaggerating? What are you talking about? What do you mean *might*?"

He handed her a glass and then sat on his bed and took a sip from his own glass. He then told her about the call from Melville's brother, everything Jacob told him, and how he has a box full of Melville's things, just in case. Prilly couldn't believe it. It was just too awful. She suddenly felt very ashamed of how she had treated Melville; she had always suspected he had a little crush on her.

As Prilly tried to process all of this shocking information, Pete got up and went to the closet. He took out a crate, which he placed on the bed. "That's it. Those are his things. Not much really, poor guy."

"May I?" Prilly asked, indicating she wanted to look in the box.

"Be my guest," Pete said.

As Prilly flipped through the papers (notes about book titles, flyers to local events, some backdated unpaid bills), Pete said, "You know, the weirdest part is something Jacob said to me. He said Melville didn't have any cousins, but that's why he always told me he was in the city. I would bump into him at the teahouse, and he'd tell me he had come into the city to see his cousin. I don't get it," he said shaking his head and taking another sip of wine.

"He was coming to see you. He must have been coming to see you and he felt embarrassed or something to say so," Prilly instantly said, now flipping through his notebooks and remembering how she had once seen him writing in one. As she heard the words come out of her mouth, she suddenly understood Melville on a deep level, and identified with him.

"Wow, you think so? Jeez. What a mindfuck. That's kind of sweet but also really sad, don't you think?" Pete asked.

"I don't know, I guess so," Prilly said. "Have you looked through these? It looks like he was writing a book or something," she continued, holding up one of the notebooks.

Pete shook his head. "I can't imagine it's very good," he said with a laugh. "I know it's terrible to say now, but Melville didn't have an original thought in his life. That's probably why he was so fascinated with me."

"Uh, huh," Prilly said, captivated by what she was reading and wanting to tell Pete he was a jerk.

"Listen, Prilly," Pete said, trying to get her attention, "I've missed you. I've missed you a lot and I think . . . "

Prilly didn't let him finish. "Pete, please. Don't. I only came because you said something horrible happened to Melville. Don't read anything else into it. I can't go there again."

"Ah, but you wouldn't have come if you didn't still have feelings for me. You know it's true. So it's silly to be stubborn about it. . . . "

"Pete, I'm going to go. You seem okay and I'm not going to do this with you. I'm not. I just can't." She got up and turned to leave. Then she paused and turned back to face Pete. "What are you going to do with those things?"

"I don't know. I guess I'll just stick them in the closet," he said, shrugging his shoulders.

"Well if you're just going to do that, do you mind if I take the notebooks? I'd like to read what he wrote. I can send them back to you if you want."

"Sure, sure, you can take them," Pete said. "You'll be disappointed, my dear, but suit yourself. Keep 'em."

Prilly removed the notebooks from the crate and headed to the front door. Pete followed her and put his hand out, shutting the door before she could walk out. She turned around, pressed firmly between Pete and the door. He leaned in to kiss her, but she turned her head. He pulled back, rejected. "I really hope Melville turns up and that he's all right," she said. Then she walked out of the apartment.

During the cab ride home, she experienced a slew of emotions. She felt sad for Melville, vindicated that Pete still wanted her, and both pride and pain at having to walk away. More than ever, the things he said and the way he said them showed her that he wasn't capable of caring about anyone except for himself. She knew that would never work for her. He was so arrogant, and for once, looking around that dingy little apartment, she couldn't quite figure out why. That night, she lay on her couch reading Melville's notebooks, which were a mix of memoir and fantasy with some mindless ramblings interspersed throughout. But there was a story in it all. It was a story about a shy and lonely man who longed to be all that he wasn't. She found it quite beautiful.

Reflection on *Low-Fat Love*

I wrote this novel to explore the concept I termed "low-fat love"—that is, settling for less in love and life and trying to pretend it's better than it is because we don't think we can get what we actually want. Years of professional and personal experiences showed me that many women settle for or stay in dissatisfying relationships because of self-esteem struggles and a learned devaluation of self. Many suffer in silence and struggle in private as they slap a happy face on in public. What does this experience look like and feel like? What psychological processes unfold? How can these patterns be broken? These were some of my guiding questions. Prilly, a fictional character, was created as a composite meant to represent countless women I had encountered over the years in interviews, classes, and my personal life. Prilly was the guide through this complex social psychological terrain.

I decided to organize the novel using a three-act structure because of its utility in building both a dramatic and a character arc. Beginning with the former, in the simplest terms, a three-act structure provides a narrative with a beginning, middle, and end. It is a way of building the dramatic arc—the inciting event and the character's struggle, escalating through rising action leading to the central conflict, and eventually the resolution. In *Low-Fat Love* the dramatic arc centers on the toxic relationship between Prilly and Pete, which reflects Prilly's own relationship with herself. The inciting incident, or first sign of trouble, occurs when Pete goes to meet Clyde, leading to the conversation in which Pete's commitment to Prilly is called into question. It's clear from Prilly's internal dialogue that this is only the beginning of their conflict. After this happens, Prilly begins to slowly unravel, leading to the inevitable confrontation when things boil over and the couple breaks up. Finally, in the end, there is the resolution or, in this case, the revelation, when Prilly accepts that the relationship with Pete will never work.

> When writing an inciting incident, it's important to make it clear that conflict is coming, but has not yet reached its peak. Leave readers wondering what's coming next and how or if things will work out.

Through the dramatic arc of the narrative, we also see the character arc—how Prilly evolves over the course of the story. This is a character's journey of self-esteem, struggle, and growth, which begins with an unraveling, until she hits bottom, and ultimately undergoes a personal transformation to bring the revelation needed to move forward.

I used three primary literary tools to construct this story: dialogue, interiority, and third-person narration. The juxtaposition of dialogue and interiority was vital for showing the disjuncture between what Prilly said versus what she was thinking and feeling. These techniques used in conjunction with each other allowed me to develop the character's unraveling by showing her psychological processes. From the second Clyde calls Pete, we hear Prilly's internal dialogue, beginning with her concern that Pete had referred to her as "a friend" and not his girlfriend. Then we see her attempt to save face or appear cool with what she says, which is contrasted with what she is thinking—her devastation that Pete is leaving her to go see another woman and her growing jealousy. We bear witness to Prilly's increasingly intense internal struggle to "stay cool" on the surface, while on the inside she's rapidly deteriorating. Readers are able to experience Prilly's undoing because her interiority is presented: we can listen to her stream of consciousness and contrast her inner thoughts to what she says and does. Representing interiority is a way of building empathetic understanding in readers. By listening in on her internal dialogue, we may be able to relate to her and feel compassion. Moreover, we can see what an unhealthy relationship looks and feels like. Prilly isn't just spinning in her mind out of nowhere, she is actively responding to what Pete says and does. In this way, we can appreciate the toll this kind of relationship takes, when one is always made to feel insecure and unsure of where things stand. Prilly's internal struggle is dialectical, that is, it occurs in relation to Pete's words and actions. Therefore, we see the effect of this form of masculinity on Prilly.

> Interiority is particularly useful for illustrating psychological processes or illustrating a disjuncture between what a character says and does and what they think and feel. Although you can create an entire internal monologue, often it's most effective to vacillate between external dialogue and interiority, both to create contrast and to allow for narrative flow. Interiority is a powerful tool for writers of social fiction, particularly when incorporating a social science perspective. A quick formatting tip: some authors don't visually distinguish external and internal dialogue; however, I recommend using italics or a different font for reader ease.

Finally, third-person narration allowed me to insert commentary into the narrative, whether that's through an analogy whereby Prilly is compared to Charlie Brown or when her feelings are summarized for readers, such as in the end when she comes to the realization that her relationship with Pete will never work.

As I reflect on *Low-Fat Love*, it occurs to me how little I knew about writing a novel at the time. It was my first effort. I have gone back and rewritten it, applying new skills, and indeed the excerpts reprinted are from the latest version, *Low-Fat Love: 10th Anniversary Edition* (Leavy, 2021d). When I originally wrote this book, I did my best and much of what ended up working was probably a result of instinct or luck. It's by no means a perfect novel, but it resonated deeply with many readers, which I believe is because it was raw and honest. People could relate to it and identify with the characters, and so it caused them to reflect on their own lives. As some of you may be faced with the task of writing your first work of fiction, I encourage you to begin from where you are, understanding that creative writing is a skill that improves over time, and when all else fails, just be honest. Authenticity resonates. Other mistakes can be forgiven.

> **SKILL-BUILDING EXERCISE** This exercise has three parts.
>
> **1.** Plotting: In earlier chapters you chose a topic and a protagonist. Based on these choices, write a general plotline for a fictional story, following a traditional three-act structure. Part 1: the set-up, including an inciting incident. Part 2: the confrontation, central conflict, or rising action. Part 3: the resolution or revelation.
>
> **2.** Story lining: Write a story line with specific scenes that get you from the beginning to the end of the plot.
>
> **3.** Writing: Use your story line to start writing, beginning with the opening scene. You can always change it later, so just start writing. If you're having trouble envisioning the opening scene, don't fret. Pick a scene from anywhere in the book that you most clearly see in your mind's eye and start writing it.

> **RETHINK YOUR RESEARCH** Based on the topic of your research, you've created a protagonist. Now you can flesh out how to transform your research project into fiction through plotting and story lining. First, using the protagonist you created, write a general plotline for a fictional work based on a traditional three-act structure. Second, write a story line with specific scenes that get you from the beginning to the end of the plot. Finally, use your story line to start writing, beginning with the opening scene. You can always change it later, so just start writing. If you're having trouble envisioning the opening scene, don't fret. Pick a scene from anywhere in the book that you most clearly see in your mind's eye and start writing it.

5 Sequels

More on Traditional Three-Act Structures

Techniques highlighted in this chapter:
- ✓ Dialogue
- ✓ Internal dialogue/interiority
- ✓ Flashbacks
- ✓ Foreshadowing
- ✓ Themes

A **sequel** is a fictional work that extends or is based on an earlier work. Typically a sequel is set after the earlier work, creating two chronological works. On the other hand, a **prequel** is a fictional work that occurs before the original story. Prequels may be created to provide more backstory to a narrative. At times an author may pen a novel, followed by a sequel and prequel, ultimately creating a trilogy (three connected works) although a trilogy may not have been planned at the outset.

There are no hard-and-fast rules for writing a sequel, although almost certainly the protagonist is the same character across the two stories. Other characters may be repeated or differ to varying degrees. The setting may also be repeated or differ, although the "story-world" remains the same. In other words, the imaginary reality in which the narrative unfolds is consistent, even if some details change (e.g., the novels take place in different geographic locations because a character has moved). Typically there is also related thematic content between an original work and a sequel, although there's a continuum on which themes reemerge and evolve. It all depends on the goal of the second book and on how closely in time the two books are set. Some authors plan sequels in advance, whereas other authors choose to continue a character's story because they feel there is more to explore or they do so as a result of positive audience response to the original work. If a work of fiction is well received, there may be incentives to continue with those characters.

Generally whatever structure is used for the original work (e.g., open form, three-act, four-act, five-act, or an alternative) should be used for the sequel. By claiming the works are linked, you set expectations for readers that need to be met. Readers will expect similarities between the two works in structure, style, tone, and, to some degree, content. In the examples that follow, both my novels *Blue* (Leavy, 2016) and *Film* (Leavy, 2020a) follow a three-act structure, just like *Low-Fat Love* discussed in the previous chapter.

Blue

I began writing *Blue* the day my daughter's biological father died after a long battle with cancer. I was home alone, trying to cope, and knew that for me the path through pain has always been creativity. So I started writing what first came to my mind, simply as a way to get through the day. I created a handwritten list of all the colors flooding my mind. They were all shades of blue. A Tori Amos song called "Garlands" was playing in the background. The song is set in New York City's Washington Square Park. Suddenly, I had symbolism and a location. I took a minor character from a previous novel, Tash Daniels, and began writing, eventually creating an outline along the way. As soon as I began writing, I knew I wanted to explore the stage in our lives when we see nothing but possibilities for ourselves as we try to figure out what we want to pursue and who we want along with us for that journey. It's only now, years later, that I realize I went back in my mind to the age I was when I met my daughter's father, when I was figuring out who I am and when the possibilities seemed limitless. Although fictional, the novel is grounded in cumulative insights from interview research, teaching, and personal observations, including my ongoing informal online communication with my students in their postgrad years.

Blue follows three roommates as they navigate life and love in their postcollege years. Tash Daniels, the former party girl, falls for deejay Aidan. Since she is always attracted to the wrong guy, what happens when the right one comes along? Jason Woo, a lighthearted model on the rise, uses the club scene as his personal playground. While he's adept at helping Tash with her personal life, how does he deal with his own life when he meets a man that defies his expectations? Penelope Brown, a reserved and earnest graduate student, slips under the radar, but she has a secret no one suspects. As the characters' stories unfold, each one is forced to confront their life choices or complacency and choose which version of themselves they want to be. *Blue* is a novel about identity, friendship, and figuring out who we are during the "in-between" phases of life and how to identify and pursue our dreams. The book shines a spotlight on the friends and lovers who become our families in the fullest sense of the word and on the search for people who "get us." These characters show how our interactions with people often bump up against backstage struggles we know nothing about. Visual art, television, and film appear as signposts throughout the narrative, providing a context for how we each come to build our sense of self in the world. In its tribute to 1980s pop culture, set against the backdrop of contemporary New York, *Blue* both celebrates and questions the ever-changing cultural landscape against which we live our stories, frame by frame.

 I selected the opening chapter as an example of the narrative exposition we expect at the beginning of a three-act structure. Primary characters are introduced, the relationships between the characters are illuminated, the setting is established, and the primary themes are foreshadowed. From the start, you are in the protagonist's head, traveling through her world.

Blue, Chapter 1

That can't be right, Tash thought, squinting again to look at the time. "Shit," she said as she reached for the alarm clock. "Damn thing never works," she mumbled while placing it back on her nightstand. *I'm gonna be late again. I should hurry.* She rolled over before slowly stretching her arms and lazily dragging herself out of bed. Stumbling to her dresser and opening the top drawer, she rifled around for underwear before heading to the bathroom.

 Twenty minutes later, wrapped in a towel after showering, she used her palm to wipe the steam from the mirror. *I look like crap. God, I hope I can cover those bags under my eyes,* she thought as she started to apply her signature black liquid eyeliner. *I'll use gray eyeshadow and make them smoky.* Realizing it must be getting late, she dried and straightened her long, dirty-blonde hair but skipped curling the ends to save time. Returning to her bedroom, she scoured her closet wondering what to wear before deciding on an off-the-shoulder, loose white tunic, a pair of skinny black jeans, and high-heeled black leather booties. Staring at herself in the mirror, she tried on four pairs of earrings, posing left and then right to fully view each option, before deciding on gold hoops. To match, she threw on her favorite gold, turquoise, and red evil-eye bracelet. *Coffee. I need coffee.*

En route to the galley kitchen, Tash stomped past her roommates' closed bedroom doors, clomping her heels without concern as to whether they were asleep. She got a bag of coffee and the nearly empty carton of milk out of the refrigerator, placed them on the counter, and opened the cupboard to get a coffee filter and her to-go tumbler, neither of which were there. She found her tumbler in the sink, dirty from the day before. *Fuck.* Turning back to focus on the coffee pot, she spotted a note sitting beside it. *There's nothing I dread first thing in the freaking morning more than these notes.*

> *Morning, Tash. Hope you didn't forget to turn the volume up on your alarm again and oversleep. I didn't want to wake you in case you had the day off. We're out of coffee filters and it's your turn to go to the store. I left my list on the back of this note. I can't cover for you this time so please go. Thanks. Have a nice day. Penelope*

Tash flipped over the note and rolled her eyes. She started to leave the kitchen when she turned back, remembering to put the milk away. *Don't want the Gestapo after me for that again,* she thought. She headed into the common room, sans coffee, and looked around. *Where did I leave my bag?* The small loveseat was overflowing with random clothing, topped with her black blazer. *Hmm. Two pairs of men's shoes under the coffee table. Jason must have met someone. Good for him, but where's my stupid bag? Ah, there you are,* spotting her black bag hiding in the corner, with her keys and sunglasses conveniently lying on top of it. She scooped them up, put her dark glasses on, and headed out, double locking the door behind her.

"Hi, Mr. Collier," she said, passing her neighbor on the stairs.

"Good morning, Miss," he replied.

Despite the morning rush, she was able to hail a cab quickly. As the cab passed Washington Square Park, she stared at the chess players, already at it for the day. Soon she drifted into thoughts of the drama the day before. *Ray was a jerk, Jason was so right. He didn't deserve me. I'm glad I ended it.* As they pulled up to Alice & Olivia, Tash rummaged through her bag for cash before giving up and surrendering her credit card to the driver.

She flew into the store, quickly heading to the backroom before Catherine could open her mouth. Tash threw her arm up and hollered, "I know, and I'm sorry. My alarm didn't go off and blah, blah, blah."

"You're half an hour late, again," Catherine called after her.

"I know, I know, and I'm sorry," Tash said, rolling her eyes. As she hung her bag and blazer on a coat hook, Catherine continued to reprimand her.

"You need to get a new alarm clock then, because I . . . "

"I'll close for you tonight, okay? You can leave early; it's fine."

"You know if you left on time you could walk here and save yourself the cab fare. You probably lose at least an hour's wages by creating a situation in which you need to take a cab. And is it even faster with the morning traffic?"

As Catherine continued, Tash muttered under her breath, "Get off my ass, you bitch," if only to make herself feel better. She took a deep breath and headed to the Keurig machine to make some much-needed coffee. She plugged it in and flipped the switch, but Catherine exclaimed, "Don't bother. It broke yesterday." Tash squeezed her eyes shut, shook her head, and took another deep breath before forcing a smile onto her face. "Great, that's just great."

* * *

"I'm going to head out now, since you're closing tonight."

"Uh huh, fine Catherine. Have a good night," Tash said while leaning on the store counter and checking her phone. She was exchanging texts with Jason, reminding him to get them on the club list that weekend.

"Make sure you change the shoes and handbags in the window display. Last season's accessories go on sale tomorrow, so the newer items should be featured in the window."

"Uh huh," Tash said, without looking up from her phone.

"Okay, well, good night."

"Night, Catherine."

An hour later, after ringing up the final customers, Tash retrieved the new handbags and shoes from the backroom. She liked working on window displays because it was a chance to be creative and put things together in unexpected ways that were sure to perplex Catherine. Tash imagined the windows as still images from a film, designed to convey a feeling as much as to display clothes. While there was a limit to what she could get away with, she pushed the bounds as much as possible. She didn't mind her job and loved working in SoHo, but window displays and the employee discount were the only aspects from which she derived genuine pleasure.

Once Tash was done putting accessories from the window onto the sale table, she gathered her things and locked up. With only a blazer on, she felt a chill. These early spring days were unusually warm but the evenings were still cold. *I should really walk home. I can't blow more money on a cab.* Desperate for a scarf, she stood on Greene Street rummaging through her slouchy leather hobo bag, which she carried everywhere despite its tendency to become a black hole in which she couldn't find anything. "Ah, there we go," she whispered as she pulled out a periwinkle scarf, which she double wrapped around her neck.

As the sky darkened, the SoHo lights seemed to shine at their brightest. Store windows screamed with flashing light bulbs, a frenetic attempt to command notice. Tash looked in the windows as she passed by, tempted by sale signs even though she was accustomed to them. These days, even New York City itself was on sale. Street vendors yearning to end their days well tried to her entice her with sunglasses and other trinkets. When she smiled and shook her head, one guy screamed, "You look like Lindsay Lohan. You're dope."

"I get that a lot," she said with a mischievous smile.

As she crossed over into the Village, the restaurants and corner cafés were already bustling with people clamoring to sit outside. After a brutal winter, New Yorkers were ready to enjoy outdoor dining again. Waiters turned on heat lamps and uncorked wine bottles amid casual conversation and bubbling laughter.

Her feet sore, she slowed her pace as she passed Washington Square Park. As day turned to night, the park was the center of the world around her. People from all walks of life appeared. The parade of artists, writers, students, homeless people, drug dealers, professors, tourists, and countless others made it the perfect microcosm of the city itself, the dream and its shadow side. She overheard a group of preppy college students talking about social justice as they passed Harold, actively trying not to notice as he set up his sleeping bag on a bench. *Jerks,* she thought. *They're such posers.*

A year earlier, Tash had twisted her ankle racing to work one morning. A barrage of f-bombs flew out of her mouth. Harold, a witness to the accident, helped her to a bench and told her not to curse.

"Are you for real?" she asked.

"It's undignified," he replied. "Do you think you can walk?"

"Uh, yeah, but not in these shoes."

They spoke for a few more minutes before she decided to stumble back to her apartment to ice her ankle and change shoes. Since that day, she'd say hi to Harold when she saw him and stopped to talk with him at least once every couple of weeks, usually bringing him a cup of coffee and sometimes a donut. Powdered sugar was his favorite.

He once started to tell his life story and she interrupted saying, "It's cool, Harold. We don't have to do this. I don't need you to explain." He seemed relieved. Since then, their conversations were usually about how they were each doing that particular day. Although routinely chased away by the police, he always returned. On this night, she just waved as she passed him.

Only half a block from her apartment, she had the horrible realization that she was supposed to get groceries. Not willing to endure a lecture from Penelope, she passed her apartment building and headed to the corner grocer. After grabbing a hand basket and making a beeline to the freezer for some ice cream, she started searching for Penelope's grocery list. As she fumbled for the list, mumbling, "Ah, where is that stupid thing?" she heard a voice say, "Maybe you'd have better luck if you shut your eyes and put your hand in."

"Huh?" she queried, looking up at the six-foot-tall guy standing before her, dressed from head to toe in black. He had bleached blonde spiky hair, high cheekbones, a strong jawline, and a piercing through his right eyebrow that she thought was simultaneously cool and disgusting.

"You know, sometimes if you're looking too hard, you can't find anything."

"Uh, yeah," she said, staring into his evergreen eyes. *Oh my God, he's seriously hot.*

"Here, tell me what you're looking for and I'll shut my eyes and stick my hand in for you."

Raising her eyebrows, she said, "How stupid do you think I am? Maybe I should just go outside and scream, 'Somebody rob me!'"

He laughed. "Fair enough, but you try it."

Tash smirked and stuck her hand into her bag without looking. "Uh huh, here it is!" she exclaimed as she pulled out the small, crumpled paper. "That's uncanny."

"Sometimes you just have to concentrate less, you know?" he said. "What's so important, anyway?"

"Oh, it's just my roommate's grocery list. She's pretty uptight so I can't screw it up. You wouldn't believe the things she writes, like 'two organic red apples and flax seed powder,' whatever the hell that is. Anyway, I should probably get back to shopping."

He smiled and waved his arm, to indicate she could pass by. With only a few aisles in the small store, Tash bumped into him again in the produce section.

"Should I even ask what that's about?" she said while giggling, looking at the twenty or more coconuts in his basket.

"Oh, these are for a party I'm deejaying for a couple of friends over at NYU."

"They're serving whole coconuts?" she asked, mystified.

He laughed. "People try to get them open. It's like a drinking game kind of thing. It's pretty funny."

"Gotcha. Do you go to NYU?"

"No, I went to school in Chicago and moved to New York after I graduated. I'm a professional deejay. I'm just doing this party as a favor."

"So, what kinds of clubs do you spin at?" she asked.

"Uh, well, tomorrow I'll be spinning at the Forever 21 store in Times Square."

She smiled. "Well, do you get a discount at least?"

He laughed. "Didn't think to ask for that. So, what's your name?"

"Natashya, but my friends call me Tash."

"I'm Aidan. Do you live around here?"

"Just a block away. I share a place with two roommates."

"Pretty awesome area to live in, good for you."

"Yeah, well we're in like the only non-restored building in the neighborhood. Don't get me wrong, I love living here and it's pretty close to my work, but we're not in one of the swanky buildings with a marble entrance. It's more like splintery wood floors and a scary old-fashioned elevator that makes me want to take the stairs."

He smiled. "What's your work?"

"I work at a couple of stores in SoHo."

"For the discount, right?" he said with a smirk.

Tash laughed. "Well, nice to meet you but I've gotta finish up and get going."

"Sure, me too. Maybe I'll see you around. If you're not busy, stop by Forever 21 tomorrow."

"I have to work."

"Well, can I maybe get your number?" he asked.

"Why don't you give me yours instead?"

"Sure, that's cool." He put his coconut-filled basket on the ground and held out his hand. "Give me your phone and I'll put it in."

"You don't want me to have to search my bag again. Here," she said, handing him the note with Penelope's grocery list. "Do you have a pen?"

Aidan smiled and pulled a red crayon out of his pocket. "Don't ask," he said as he wrote his number on the little paper. "Here," he said handing it to her. "See ya."

"See ya," she said.

When she casually glanced around the store a few minutes later, he was gone. She brought her basket to the checkout. The cashier asked, "Did you find everything you needed?"

"Yeah, yeah I did."

* * *

Her feet aching and her arms overloaded, Tash felt like she was going to drop by the time she made it home. She dumped her handbag and keys on the entryway floor and swung the shopping bags onto the kitchen counter. She opened her new box of popcorn and stuck a packet in the microwave before putting the rest of the groceries away. She giggled to herself, thinking about the coconuts filling Aidan's basket. *I wonder if Jason is home.*

Tash met Jason Woo at a club a few years earlier. She was having trouble getting past the bouncers when Jason came to her rescue. His modeling career was just starting to take off thanks to landing a gig as Calvin Klein's first Asian male model. Both sarcastic and carefree, they bonded immediately and moved in together as soon as Tash graduated from college. Though they had a hard time looking out for themselves, they did a remarkable job of looking out for each other.

Tash was so lost in thought about Aidan's coconuts that she didn't hear Jason approaching.

"Hey," Jason said from the doorway.

"Oh, hey." She tossed him a bag of coffee. "Stick that in the fridge." As he put the coffee away, Tash said, "This too," and flung the loaf of bread.

"I can't believe you actually went shopping. Did Pen leave you one of her famous notes?"

"Yup," she said just when the microwave beeped. "Is she in her room studying?"

"She's not here. I think she had dinner plans with her study group or something."

"Seriously? She's unbelievable, making me do all this when she's not even here," she said as she opened the popcorn bag. Steam burned her hand and caused her to drop the bag on the counter. "Fuck," she mumbled.

"How is it you never learn not to open it that way?" Jason asked facetiously. "Here, I got it," he said. He grabbed a bowl from the cupboard and emptied the bag for her.

"You know if you leave it in the bag it's one less dish to wash. That's why I do that."

"Since when do you ever wash the dishes anyway?" he rebuffed, as he ate a handful of her popcorn.

"I don't know why she made me go to the store if she wasn't even gonna be home," Tash said as she threw the two empty grocery bags in the garbage.

"I know you can't relate, but some people actually plan ahead. She probably wanted breakfast."

"Oh, right, like you plan ahead," Tash jabbed, tossing a jar of maraschino cherries.

"You're lucky I caught that. What is it with you and these things?" he asked, sticking them in the door of the refrigerator.

"You know I love them. I can't help it," she said. "But listen, I kind of met a guy. I met him at the store while I was getting Pen's crap, so maybe it was meant to be."

"You met a guy? Ah, do tell," he prodded.

"Well from the looks of things this morning, I'm guessing you also met a guy, so you tell first." She opened the refrigerator and grabbed two cans of Diet Coke.

"Some lighting guy from the shoot. I kicked him out this morning."

"You're such a slut. Must be hard to be so irresistible," Tash bemused.

Jason smiled. "You would know. Come on, let's go curl up on my bed and you can tell me all about the guy you met. I hope he's better than Ray. I'm eating half this popcorn, by the way," he said, taking a fistful and heading to his room.

"Hey, that's my dinner!"

Reflection on *Blue*

As the primary goal of this chapter is to introduce readers to the protagonist and her relationship to other characters, I employed three techniques: interiority, dialogue, and flashbacks. Interiority is used, beginning with the opening words, to bring readers into Tash's mind. We get a sense from the start that she's at least somewhat vain, insensitive to her roommates, and unmotivated to do well at her job. Through interiority we also see how she reacts to different people and situations. We are exposed to her feelings. For example, we learn Tash gets annoyed by her roommate Penelope, that she's recently ended a romantic relationship, and that she's attracted to Aidan as soon as they meet. We learn these tidbits about the character through her own thoughts. Dialogue is used to show how she interacts with different people and to illustrate the nature of different relationships. For example, dialogue or unfolding action shows her frustration with her boss and her job as well as the close relationship she has with her roommate and bestie, Jason. Finally by using a flashback scene that recounts how she met Harold, the homeless man she befriended, we get to see a different facet of this character, her compassionate side. The combination of these techniques shows readers up-front a multidimensional view of Tash—some of what may be perceived as both her positive and negative traits. She's flawed and relatable.

> "Meet cutes" are scenes in which romantic couples meet for the first time, generally in a humorous or memorable way. Aidan's basket full of coconuts and the conversation that ensued, ending with him writing down his phone number with a crayon, is an example. This unusual meeting even leads to Aidan being called "Coconut Boy" in later parts of the novel. When writing a romantic story line, a meet cute can help quickly bring readers into the relationship. Spend some time thinking about a fun or offbeat way your characters can meet.

A secondary goal of this chapter is to hint at the thematic content of the novel. In other words, there is foreshadowing. This is a story about figuring out who we are before our life choices feel "locked"[1] and identifying the dreams we wish to pursue. Tash's attitude toward her retail job is evidenced throughout this chapter, beginning with her lackadaisical response to realizing she's running late and later in her interactions with her boss. Clearly she's frustrated and uninspired. We see a glimmer of what brings her joy and fulfillment when she's arranging store window displays, imagining them as stills from a film. Later readers learn Tash's passion is filmmaking and she has a film studies degree from New York University. Her failure to pursue her true passion, and learning to confront that failure, is ultimately central to the narrative.

Film

Film is a sequel to *Blue* that takes place a few years later and follows Tash and two other women, who moved to Los Angeles to pursue their dreams, each in a creative industry. Tash has been trying in earnest to be a filmmaker. Her short film was rejected from festivals, she has a stack of rejected grant proposals, and she lost her internship at a studio when her boss sexually harassed her, forcing her to take a job as a personal shopper. Lu K is a hot deejay who is slowly working her way up the club scene, but no one is doing her any favors. Fiercely independent, she's at a loss when she meets Paisley, a woman who captures her heart. Monroe Preston is the glamorous wife of a Hollywood studio head. As a teenager she moved to LA in search of a "big life," but now she wonders if the reality measures up to the fantasy. When a man in their circle finds sudden fame, each of these women is catapulted on a journey of self-discovery. As the characters' stories unfold, each is forced to confront how her past has shaped her fears and to choose how she wants to live in the present. *Film* is a novel about the underside of dreams, the struggle to find internal strength, the power of art, and what it truly means to live a "big life." What does the pursuit of happiness look and feel like for women in the context of #MeToo experiences? Frequently shown bathed in the glow of the silver screen, the characters in *Film* show us how the arts can reignite the light within. In its tribute to popular culture, set against the backdrop of Tinseltown, *Film* celebrates how the art we make and consume can shape our stories, scene by scene.

 The first chapter of a sequel generally brings you up-to-date with the protagonist—where they are now, what they're doing, how much time has passed, what characters from the original novel are still in their life, and what new characters are being introduced. All of this action occurs in the first chapter of *Film*. I have chosen not to use that opening chapter as the exemplar for two reasons. First, for those who have not yet read *Blue*, I don't want to spoil anything. Second, in Chapter 4 I took you through one character's journey at different moments (Prilly in *Low-Fat Love*). Instead of using a similar example, I've chosen Chapter 10 from *Film*, which focuses on building thematic content. The chapter is an illustration of how to build one theme through multiple characters across books. In *Blue*, characters struggle to identify and grab hold of their dreams as they linger in in-between spaces. This theme intensifies and moves forward in *Film*, in which the women characters are actively pursuing their dreams, but stumbling along the way as they are forced to deal with sexual harassment and other gendered experiences that derail them.

The following chapter centers on Monroe Preston. Now in her 40s, she came to LA as a teenager to pursue a career as a model and actress, dying her hair platinum blonde and changing her name. Eventually she gives up those pursuits, marries a wealthy studio head, and lives what many may consider an enviable life. However, she's been depressed and unable to sleep for weeks. She fears her life is slipping away. She becomes consumed by memories of growing up poor in the middle of nowhere, her desire for a sparkly and glamorous life in entertainment, and her complex relationship with her now deceased mother. Monroe longed to be nothing like her, a lonely seamstress who raised Monroe as a single parent. To combat her depression and fatigue, her husband suggests a visit to their vacation house.

Film, Chapter 10

"Monroe, is there anything you'd like me to put in the car?" Bill called from the bedroom.

Monroe stared in the bathroom mirror, wondering if the dark circles under her eyes were as pronounced as she feared, or if they were like her heartbeat, louder in her own mind. She took a deep breath before responding, "No thank you, darling. Henry already loaded my small travel bag and my books."

"I need to make a quick call. I'll meet you at the car."

"Be down in a minute."

Even that brief exchange depleted her energy, so she sat perfectly still, taking deep, purposeful breaths. She plucked a tube of concealer off the vanity, rubbed the porcelain-colored goop on her fingertip, and gently dabbed it under each eye. She sat for another moment, vacantly gazing at the mirror before sauntering into her bedroom to fetch her beige Hermès handbag and oversized, black Chanel sunglasses. At the last minute, she rifled through her nightstand and removed an unopened prescription for valium. With the bottle tucked safely in her handbag, Monroe headed out. She stopped at her beloved Warhol, almost involuntarily, and cocked her head as if trying to see the brightly colored image from a new perspective. *Marilyn, I read something you wrote, something about how you felt life coming closer. Had it been further? Had you been removed from your* own life? Is that what Mr. Warhol saw? Is that what he was trying to show us?*

Her daydream was interrupted when Bill called from the bottom of the staircase. "We should get on the road before the traffic picks up."

She smiled ever so slightly at the painting, slipped on her sunglasses, and hollered, "Coming, darling."

* * *

Bill turned north onto the 101, flipping through the stations on the radio.

"Oh, leave that on," Monroe said, as Billie Holiday's voice oozed through the speakers.

"Looks like an easy ride today," he said.

"You should have taken the driver so you could relax."

"It's my only chance to drive. If I had my way, we'd be in one of the convertibles."

"Oh Bill, you know the wind and sun are too much for me."

"That's why I leave one of them at the ranch house. We can just do a short, local drive when we're there. It's an excuse for you to put your hair up in one of those silk scarves I bought you in Paris."

"Mmhmm," Monroe sighed.

"Maybe you should try to take a nap. It's been weeks since you've slept properly. I don't remember you suffering like this since before we got married, after your. . . ." he trailed off.

"Yes, I know."

"Back then, your doctor prescribed something. Maybe. . . ."

Monroe interrupted. "Yes, I already got something, just in case."

"Hopefully you won't need it. A change of scenery will do you good. Riding always knocks you out, and the horses will be happy to see you too."

She turned toward him and smiled faintly. "I think you're right, darling. Perhaps I'll close my eyes for a bit."

"When we get to Ventura, should I stop at that produce stand you like?" Bill asked. "We could get greens for your smoothies and maybe some melon for breakfast."

"All right," she muttered, her eyelids becoming heavier. As Billie Holiday warbled her last note, Monroe shut her eyes.

I should remember to get kale and spinach. Oh, and cucumbers. I always forget the cucumbers. Bill wants melon. Perhaps they'll have nice cantaloupe. He loves cantaloupe. Suspended somewhere between sleeping and waking, her thoughts drifted to the supermarket where she worked at as a teenager. She remembered the day she quit, at the age of sixteen, as if it had just happened.

Her twenty-two-year-old manager, Tom, a tall, skinny man with dark hair and sparse stubble on his short chin, called her over the store intercom.

"Jenny Anne to the stockroom."

She headed straight to the stockroom, glad to have a break from bagging groceries, a job that made time move slower than the little turtles Lauren raced with her brother. Tom was already in the small, dank room, holding a clipboard. A crate of honeydew melons sat atop a stack of boxes.

"These melons need to be shelved," he said.

"Sure thing," she replied, wriggling past him in the cramped space. She placed her hand on a melon when she heard the clipboard drop onto the small table beside them. Suddenly, she felt him standing behind her, not a centimeter separating them.

"Those melons should be ripe," he said, his voice lower than usual.

"Uh huh," she mumbled.

He placed his hand on the melon she was touching, his body now pressed against her.

"You've been here for almost a year, right?" he asked softly. "Feel that melon. When something's ripe, it starts to smell different. When you bite into it, the sweetness drips from your mouth."

Her heart thumping, she said, "I'm all set here. I got it on my own."

"You sure you don't need my help?" he whispered, still pressed firmly against her.

"I'm all set," she replied, trying to control her shaking.

He stepped back. "When you're done with those, you can go on your break."

She inhaled, holding her breath until she was certain he was gone. She shelved all the melons, collected her backpack from her locker, and walked out of the store as if she was taking her break. She never went back, not even to get her last paycheck.

By the time she got home, tears were streaming down her face. She cleaned herself up before her mother got home from work, not wanting to upset her after a long day and afraid she might blame her "attention-getting" appearance for the incident. At dinner, she casually announced she quit her job because it had nothing to do with what she wanted to do in life. For weeks, she and her mother argued about it, her mother insisting "life isn't just made up of things we like." Lauren was the only person she confided in. After that, whenever her mother sent her to the grocery store, she took two buses to go to the store two towns over.

Every night, as she lay in bed counting the Day-Glo shooting stars on her ceiling, she dreamt of a life far away from minimum wage, managers, and buses. Sometimes she'd picture herself on the cover of Vogue and she'd imagine Tom, old and ugly, bagging groceries and looking at stacks of magazines adorned with her face.

* * *

As they pulled away from the produce stand, Bill turned the radio back on. Sinatra came through the speakers. "Ah, this is perfect for the scenic part of the drive," Bill said.

Monroe smiled. "You're so old-fashioned. I do love that about you."

Bill laughed. "I've been blessed with good taste."

Monroe giggled. "I love the coastal part of the trip." She gazed past Bill, the deep blue water of the Pacific glistening in the sun. "The water in California always sparkles," she said softly.

Bill turned the music up and Monroe watched the water as if it were a film where the past and present met. Her husband provided the soundtrack. Her eyelids once again became heavy, but she fought to keep them open.

It always sparkles, she thought. *I'll never forget the first time I saw the Pacific. Vast and glorious, just like I imagined my future would be.*

She landed in LA with less than a thousand dollars in the bank and everything she owned crammed into two suitcases. She had hustled, mailing her semi-professional headshots to various modeling and talent agencies, the latter offering no response. However, she had meetings arranged with three modeling agencies and was told if she was signed, they would help her get settled and send her on go-sees to clients right away. Confident that she could make big things happen for herself, she ignored her bank balance and hailed a cab at LAX. When the cabdriver asked, "Where to?" she handed him a slip of paper with the address of a cheap motel she had booked. He warned her, "Be careful. That's a rough area."

"That's okay. I won't be there long. Oh, and sir, can you drive by the Pacific? I've never seen it before."

"It's out of your way and will cost you more."

"That's okay. Please take the longer route."

* * *

When the Prestons arrived at their home away from home, they were promptly greeted by their housekeeper, who ran outside to help them. Bill handed her the cardboard box overflowing with fresh produce.

"Oh my, these berries are beautiful," she said. "I'll get these into the house right away."

"Thank you," Bill said, as he retrieved Monroe's bag from the trunk. "Feeling better? You dozed off in the car."

"Yes, a bit better."

"Shall we head inside?"

Monroe nodded. "I think after we settle in, I'll go to the stables, see the horses. Perhaps I'll go for a short ride."

Monroe changed into her riding clothes in her bedroom. She noticed the small, framed photograph of her mother on her dresser. Her mother was young and uncharacteristically wearing a party dress. It was Monroe's favorite photo. She picked it up and smiled. "Oh Mama, you were beautiful. Strange how you spent your life making party dresses for other women, but never for yourself. You never did care much for fancy clothes or makeup, but you didn't need any of that. I'm sorry I thought you were plain or simple. You weren't, were you?"

She gently placed the frame back on the dresser and sat on the edge of the bed, thinking about the day she called her mother boasting she'd been signed to a modeling agency.

"Mama, I don't understand why you aren't more excited."

"I told you, I'm happy for you if this is what you want."

"They set me up with an apartment with a bunch of other girls. They think I'd be good at print work, and I have go-sees all week."

"Go . . . ?"

"Go-sees, Mama. They're like auditions."

"The thought of you parading around for them and being judged—judged on your God-given body. . . ."

Monroe rolled her eyes. "It's not like that, not really. Besides, if I book some jobs, I'll be able to take another stab at talent agencies, maybe try my hand at acting."

"I just don't know how anyone could be happy like that, being rejected all the time."

"Mama, did you ever think that some people just are happy, and even if they're not, they're trying to be?" After a long silence, Monroe changed the subject. "What about you, Mama?"

"Oh, well, I'm fine. I'm the same."

"How's work?"

"The same as always."

"Have you gone to play cards at Elaine's?"

"I've been too tired." She paused for a moment. "Jenny Anne, we should hang up. This call will be very expensive for you."

"Maybe someday we won't have to worry about that. I'll call you next week."

"Call after seven when it's less expensive."

"Yes, Mama."

"And Jenny Anne, if you're happy, *truly* happy, that's all a person can hope for, I suppose."

"I'll call next week. Wish me luck. Bye, Mama."

All these years later, Monroe could recall every detail of that conversation. *Was dressmaking in that small town really your ideal life? I remember the stacks of unpaid bills, and you, sitting alone every night, eating reheated casserole and watching game shows. Weekends spent cleaning the house or doing odd jobs. Oh, I wish I knew what your dreams had been. You must have had some, even if you held onto them tightly. Or was it that you let them go too easily?* Her thoughts shifted to her mother's words about happiness: "If you're happy, *truly* happy, that's all a person can hope for." She began to wonder about her tone. She tried to remember how she sounded. *Were you mournful? Was I too preoccupied to truly hear you? Oh Mama, were you ever happy? If you were, when did your happiness end? When did life slip farther away?*

* * *

Luke, the stablehand, had prepared Monroe's favorite horse, Captain, in case she wanted to go for a ride. As she mounted the beautiful animal, his coat the color of dark chocolate with creamy white splotches along his gait, she whispered, "Oh Captain, how I've missed you."

"I took him out for a walk so he's ready for whatever you have in mind. I'll be here when you get back," Luke said.

Monroe nodded and then gently pressed on her horse. He began walking. There was little that brought Monroe the peace and joy she felt with her horses. She'd spent twenty-five years searching for meaning in religion, spirituality, astrology, mythology, self-help, and countless fads that had quickly come and gone, but she felt most centered when she was riding. It cleared her mind. But today, she couldn't focus on the horse, the breeze, or the sunshine. She couldn't quiet her mind. She began to wonder why she felt out of sorts these past few weeks, unsettled, and outside of the moment.

Bill adores me. Our lives are perfect. I have more freedom and glamour than I ever could have envisioned. What's wrong with me? Her mother's words came barreling into her mind. *"Glamour alone isn't a goal. It isn't a life."* She remembered when she called her mother to announce her engagement and the argument that ensued.

"Why are you always so negative? You're never happy for me."

"That isn't true. I just don't want to see you throw your life away. You're too young, you barely know him, and my God, Jenny Anne, he's too old for you."

"Stop being so provincial. He's not old, he's accomplished."

"And what will you accomplish in your life?"

"Do you know how many girls would kill to marry someone like Bill? Do you know how lucky I am?"

"You need time to find out who you are and what you can do for yourself. There will always be men who want to take care of a girl as pretty as you."

"Then why were you alone your whole life?" she shrieked. "Working till your fingers were raw, sitting alone at home and crying at night. Don't you think I heard you, whimpering, crying yourself to sleep?"

No response. When what seemed like an eternity had passed, Monroe softened her voice. "I'm sorry, Mama. You know I'm grateful for everything you did for me. I just want you to be happy for me. We're different, that's all."

"Jenny Anne, I hope you find what you're looking for. Call me next week."

"Bill is gonna buy your airline ticket for the wedding. He'll take care of everything. Don't forget, it's just a couple of months away."

"I'll talk to you next week."

"Bye, Mama."

Embarrassed by what she had said and preoccupied with planning a whirlwind wedding, she didn't call her mother for three weeks. When they finally spoke, her mother was quieter than usual, distant. Things that would usually provoke an argument got no reaction at all. Her mother's response to everything was, "that's nice," which was how she always spoke to others, but never to Monroe. Feeling guilty, Monroe assumed her change in demeanor was because of the hurtful words she had spoken weeks earlier.

Three days later, a police officer called to inform her that her mother had been killed in a car accident. Her car veered off the road, slamming into a tree. Monroe was devastated. Instead of flying her mother out to California, Monroe and Bill flew in for the funeral. After the service, she hosted mourners in her mother's home. The next-door neighbor, Elaine, walked over and hugged Monroe tightly. Elaine and her mother sometimes stopped at each other's homes for coffee, to play cards, or with a bowl of soup if one or the other was sick.

"I'm just so sorry, Jenny Anne. I always knew of your mother's troubles, but if I had thought...."

Monroe's eyes widened. "What are you saying, Elaine? It was a car accident."

Elaine took Monroe's hands. "It was a clear night and there were no skid marks. No other cars. You've always been such a firecracker that you kept her going, kept the flicker of fight alive in her. But once you were grown.... I'm sure you knew... she always had such a sadness about her. She..."

Monroe squeezed her hands and released. "Thank you for coming."

Monroe didn't sleep for weeks. Bill suggested postponing the wedding, but she refused, saying, "Life is too short." He couldn't argue.

As she rode her horse, the afternoon sun beating on her face, she thought about every word her mother spoke in those final phone calls, trying to compare them to all the words she had spoken before. The words were like an avalanche threatening to overtake her mind. She squeezed her calves and heels and her horse began to gallop. *"You need to find out who you are. Glamour alone isn't a goal. Fancy dresses and parties don't make people happy. Life will disappoint you. You look like tinsel sparkling under twinkly lights."* Desperate to outrun the avalanche, she applied more pressure and screamed, "Go, Captain." He began galloping at full speed, the wind pushing against her skin, pushing against the words.

Reflection on *Film*

Interiority, dialogue, and flashbacks, the same tools used in *Blue*, are used in the sequel to reveal the theme of the book (e.g., women pursuing their dreams in the context of #MeToo experiences). For each of the three primary characters, readers observe how their dreams took hold, what obstacles were in their way, how their identities developed in relation to those pursuits and challenges, and how they struggle to make peace with their choices so they can move forward.

In the preceding example, we begin with a glimpse into Monroe's fatigued mind-set. She's depressed and suffering an identity crisis, thoughts we learn as she interacts with an Andy Warhol painting of her idol. Soon we see how Monroe's experiences as a teenager and young adult continue to have ripple effects years later. Flashbacks allow us to understand how sexual harassment as a teenager impacts a woman throughout her life and are useful because they allow for scenic writing—the action is unfolding in real time, although it occurred in the past. We can see and feel a character's past experiences and contextualize them within the present. For example, a trip to a produce stand reminds Monroe of when her boss sexually harassed her decades earlier, the profound effect that had on her life, including her bumpy relationship with her mother, and how experiences like that, in part, shaped her dreams. As the chapter progresses, through a combination of interiority, dialogue, and flashbacks, we learn more about Monroe's move to LA, her struggles with her mother, the growing inner rumblings that she's not happy, and the circumstances around her mother's death. Parallels are drawn between her mother's melancholic state of mind and her own. Ultimately the recurring, layered theme centers on what the pursuit of dreams looks like and feels like for women.

SKILL-BUILDING EXERCISE Dialogue and interior dialogue help us develop characters while moving the plot forward. Write a conversation between your protagonist and another character. Include interior dialogue, which if you're stuck, can be done before or after the conversation in order to show what a character thinks or feels going into the conversation or as a result of the interaction. If you're having trouble coming up with an idea, show the conversation that ensues when the two characters first meet (which could even be written as a flashback).

RETHINK YOUR RESEARCH Create another character who is important in your protagonist's story and is based on your research participants. Again the character may be based on one participant or may be a composite based on an aggregate of data. If your research doesn't involve participants, use a literature review to wholly imagine a character. Once you've created your second character, write a conversation between both characters. Include interior dialogue, which if you're stuck, can be done before or after the conversation in order to show what a character thinks or feels going into the conversation or as a result of the interaction.

NOTES

1. I'm not in any way suggesting that our life choices become "locked" at any phase—it's never too late to change course and indeed change our lives. I'm merely noting that people may begin to feel as if their life is set and the possibilities for change are shrinking (e.g., after marriage, having children, or establishing a career).

6 Series and Open Form Structures

> Techniques highlighted in this chapter:
> - ✓ Characterization
> - ✓ Foreshadowing
> - ✓ Themes, style, and tone
> - ✓ Juxtaposition
> - ✓ Story line/scenes/pacing
> - ✓ Metaphor
> - ✓ Symbolism
> - ✓ Endings/closure
> - ✓ Epilogues
> - ✓ Titles

Sometimes fiction writers create multiple linked works, beyond the two works that comprise a novel and sequel. Common variations are trilogies, serials, and novel sequences. **Trilogies** are three connected works that generally share repeating characters, settings, and/or themes. Typically, a trilogy follows a protagonist across one character arc, unfolding over three novels. They are usually read in order. **Novel sequences** refer to several novels that share the same characters, settings, and/or themes but have their own contained story line. Thus these novels can be read as stand-alone books. However, there are overarching themes or narrative arcs that emerge when the novels in the sequence are read chronologically. Finally, **serials** are longer works that follow the same character or characters but are divided into installments. There may be one narrative that is told across several stories or books.

It's important to note that while the term **series** has multiple meanings in the world of publishing, it is also commonly used to describe a collection of more than three novels following the same character, whether in one large narrative or several stand-alone narratives. In practice, the term "novel sequences" is rarely used. The more familiar or popular term "serial" or "series" is generally applied when writers produce novels that follow the same characters across more than three books, even when they can be read as independent novels and there are overarching themes and narrative arcs. Accordingly, in my discussion of the Tess Lee and Jack Miller novels, I use the terms serial and series, although these books can easily be viewed as a novel sequence.

When writing multiple connected works, it's important to maintain the same writing style, which readers will become familiar with and come to expect. Connected works of fiction need to be consistent for readers, not just in terms of content, but also in tone and style. For instance, if interiority is used in one novel, it should be used in all of them. In the case of the Tess Lee and Jack Miller novels, the stories unfold in real time, solely through dialogue and interaction. I did not use devices I've used in the past, such as flashbacks or interiority, because I wanted readers to experience the characters as they experience each other. Whatever choices you make when writing a trilogy or serial, they should be consistent.

While the novels excerpted in previous chapters follow a three-act structure, the Tess Lee and Jack Miller novels use an open form structure. An **open form structure** does not follow prescribed patterns and is not organized in a specific way. The narrative flows freely, chapter to chapter, and is not broken down into parts. Although this openness allows the story to develop in its own unique way, as with all narrative fiction, there is generally a beginning, middle, and end, which consist of the set-up, confrontation, and resolution. An open form structure may be used for one fictional work or multiple works (as discussed in this chapter). So even if you're only interested in writing one work of fiction, the extracts reprinted in this chapter model the organic nature of an open form structure grounded primarily in scenic writing.

Celestial Bodies:
The Tess Lee and Jack Miller Novels

Celestial Bodies (Leavy, 2022) is a collection that includes the books *Shooting Stars, Twinkle, Constellations, Supernova, North Star,* and *Stardust.* Although the work is a serial whose narrative arc ultimately reveals a larger journey, each book was written as a stand-alone novel and can be read on its own. This serial is an exploration of love—in all forms—romance, friendship, patriotism, love of art, and most important, love of ourselves.

Tess Lee and Jack Miller's love story is the heart of this serial. Tess Lee is a world-famous novelist and philanthropist. Her inspirational books explore people's innermost struggles and the human need to believe that there is light at the end of the tunnel. Despite her extraordinary success, she's been unable to find personal happiness and is in the lifelong process of recovery from childhood abuse. Jack Miller is a federal agent. After spending decades immersed in a violent world, a residue remains. He's dedicated everything to his job, leaving nothing for himself. He also struggles with grieving the death from leukemia of his 4-year-old daughter, whom he didn't know until she was on her deathbed. These are two innately good people who have sacrificed in service of others, and found little for themselves, until they find each other. There's a saying that "hurt people hurt people," but Tess and Jack show us that hurt people can love each other in extraordinary ways. In essence, the couple, along with their close friends, model what love looks like in action.

The other central relationship in the series is the deep friendship between Tess and Omar. While Jack is the love of Tess's life, Omar is her soul mate, her chosen family. They met on orientation day during freshman year of college when they wandered onto a football field and shared their dreams. Tess was estranged from her childhood family due to the abuse she suffered, and Omar's family severed all ties when he came out as gay. They decided to be each other's family. Since her first novel was released, Omar has been calling Tess by the nickname "Butterfly" for reasons revealed near the end of *Shooting Stars.* Throughout the series, his use of the name Butterfly signifies their close and special relationship. Omar is wickedly funny and the two routinely joke around and tease one another. This relationship is important for many reasons, not the least of which is challenging the pervasive idea in popular culture that our "soul mate" is a lover, when in fact, for many, that person may be a best friend.

Each novel in the series explores love and another topic, and each has its own theme. *Shooting Stars* looks at love and healing, explaining themes of darkness and light. *Twinkle* looks at love and doubt; its theme is the relationship between the small part and the greater whole. The theme of *Constellations* is intimacy, and it focuses on love and family. *Supernova* explores love and trust, returning to the themes of darkness and light. *North Star* explores love and commitment through a theme of and letting go and living in color. *Stardust,* not discussed in detail in this book, explores love and faith through a theme of acceptance. Together these books are an exploration of love—a grand love letter to love itself.

When writing connected works of fiction, it's advisable to consider how the titles relate to one another. In this case, I selected a celestial theme. The meaning of each title is revealed near the end of each book and is intricately linked to the theme of that particular story.

Selecting chapters as exemplars from this serial was challenging. Each novel begins with a scene featuring just Tess and Jack because this is their love story; each novel ends with an epilogue that concludes with Tess speaking, because she is our heroine. Each novel also includes an excerpt from one of Tess's books, which reflects and synthesizes themes in the novel; scenes at Shelby's Bar where this group of friends or "chosen family" regularly shares stories and laughs; and a fluid mix of both dramatic and/or traumatic scenes as well as lighter scenes filled with humor. All of this material needed to be represented in the five chapters I selected. Furthermore, the central relationships needed to be covered: Tess and Jack, Tess and Omar, the entire friendship group, and minor characters. The thematic content of each book also needed to be present in the chosen selection. Add to this, from a writer's perspective, I wanted to share extracts of different lengths and scopes, so I could offer commentary on how one approaches contained scenes versus sprawling chapters. Finally, I wanted to select chapters that could be understood and even enjoyed, if one has not read the novel. In short, selecting chapters was a bigger task than I had imagined. I didn't necessarily pick my favorite chapter from each book, but rather chapters that in their totality reflect these different aspects of the series and allow for illustration of the different aspects of literary writing reviewed in Chapter 3.

Shooting Stars

The night Tess and Jack meet, their connection is palpable. She examines the scars on his body and says, "I've never seen anyone whose outsides match my insides." The two embark on an epic love story that asks the questions: What happens when people truly see each other? Can unconditional love change the way we see ourselves? Their friends are along for the ride: Omar, Tess's sarcastic best friend, who mysteriously calls her Butterfly; Joe, Jack's friend from the Bureau, who understands the sacrifices he's made; and Bobby and Gina, Jack's younger friends who never fail to lighten the mood. *Shooting Stars* is a novel about walking through our past traumas, moving from darkness to light, and the ways in which love from lovers, friends, or the art we experience heals us.

What follows is the opening chapter of *Shooting Stars*. There was no choice but to select this chapter. After all, this is Tess and Jack's love story, and so it's important to see how it all began.

Shooting Stars, Chapter 1

"How's your son doing in school?" Tess asked the bartender.

"Really well. He especially loves the history course he's taking."

A man came in and sat two stools down from Tess. They looked at each other and smiled in acknowledgment.

"Hey, Jack. The usual?" the bartender asked.

Jack nodded. "Please."

Tess continued chatting with the bartender as he served Jack a bottle of beer. "The humanities are so important. It's a shame they're undervalued," she said.

"You're the expert," the bartender replied.

Just then, a different man sidled up to Tess. "You have the most beautiful brown eyes," he said.

"Do I?" she asked.

"And the way your hair flows all the way down your back. You know what they say about dirty blondes?"

"I don't think you should finish that sentence," Tess said.

"I've been watching you. Can I buy you a drink?" he asked.

"No, thank you," she replied.

"Come on, just one drink. I'm a nice guy."

"No, thank you," she said, turning away.

The "nice guy" opened his mouth to protest, but Jack stood up with an imposing air and said, "The lady said no."

The man snorted and walked away.

"Thank you," Tess said, staring straight into his sea-colored eyes.

"Don't mention it. I did feel a little sorry for him, though. You are beautiful and I can't blame him for taking a shot."

Tess smiled and pulled out the stool next to her. "Please, scooch over. Let me buy your drink."

He smiled and took the seat next to her. "My name is Tess Lee," she said.

"Jack Miller," he replied. "But it's on me. Yours looks nearly empty. What are you having?"

"Sparkling water. I don't drink. It's just a personal choice," she replied.

"Another sparkling water for my new friend," Jack said to the bartender. "So, Tess, what brings you here by yourself?"

"I was supposed to meet my best friend, Omar, but he had a last-minute emergency. His partner, Clay, was pulled over tonight and it became an incident."

"What was he pulled over for?" Jack asked.

"Being Black," Tess replied. "Clay is a surgeon and was on his way home from the hospital. He was pulled over for no reason and harassed. It's happened to him before. Once, he was on his way to an emergency at the hospital, and he was detained even after he showed his hospital ID. It's egregious. Anyway, I told Omar to stay home with him. They need time together to process and decompress. Omar understands this kind of experience, being of Middle Eastern descent. I was already in a cab on my way here, so I decided to come anyway. I moved to DC from LA about six months ago and I don't have that much of a life yet, I suppose. And you?"

"My friends ditched me. We usually get together on Friday nights at a different bar, but they all had to stay late at work. This place is right down the block from my apartment."

"So, what do you do?" she asked.

"I'm a federal agent with the Bureau, working in counterterrorism. I joined the military right out of high school, Special Forces. I was in the field, often deep undercover, until about a year ago, when I took a desk job as the head of my division."

"Wow, you're like the real-life Jack Bauer. You even look a little like him, with that whole rugged, handsome, hero thing you have going on," she said.

He blushed. "I promise you I'm no Jack Bauer, even on my best day. People thought that character was so tragic, but the real tragedy is that Jack Bauer doesn't exist and you're stuck with guys like me."

She smiled. "What made you choose that line of work?"

"My parents raised me and my siblings to value community, to be patriotic. My father was in the military and then became a firefighter. The idea of service always seemed important. I wanted to serve my country, to protect people. It's hard to explain, but when I see someone innocent being threatened, I'm willing to do whatever is necessary to protect them. I know it sounds cliché, but I feel like it's my purpose in life."

"That's noble," she said.

He shook his head. "The lived reality often isn't. When you spend most of your life in the abyss, it gets pretty dark."

"A residue remains, right?" she asked.

He looked at her intently, a little surprised. "Yes, exactly."

"I understand. You convince yourself it's all been for something that matters more than you do, that whatever part of yourself you sacrificed was worth it, because it simply has to be."

He looked at her as if she had read his innermost thoughts. "Yes," he said softly. "Tell me, what do you do?"

"I'm a novelist."

"What are your books about?" he asked.

"That's a hard question to answer. I guess I wanted to write about everything: What it means to live a life, why it's so hard, and how it could be easier. To walk people through the darkness, in a way. Perhaps my goals were too lofty, and in that respect, each book fails more spectacularly than the one before."

The bartender smirked.

Tess wistfully said, "Maybe reality can never live up to our dreams."

They continued talking, completely engrossed with one another. Two hours later, Jack said, "I live nearby. Do you want to come over for a cup of coffee?"

Tess looked him straight in his warm eyes. "I'd love to."

Jack threw some money down on the bar to cover both tabs. The bartender said, "Ms. Lee, are you sure you're all right? I can call you a cab."

"You're very kind, but I'm fine. Thank you."

Jack opened the door and held it for Tess. "Do you know the bartender?"

"Just met him tonight," she replied.

"Down this way," Jack said, taking her hand as if it were completely natural. They approached a homeless man on the corner asking for money. Tess walked right up to him, pulled a twenty-dollar bill from her pocket, and handed it to him. She held his hand as she passed the bill, looked in his eyes, and said, "Be well."

As they walked away, Jack said, "That was really sweet, but you should be more careful."

"I trust my instincts," she replied.

When they arrived at Jack's small apartment, he took her coat. She glanced around and noticed the walls were completely bare. "How long have you lived here?" she asked.

"About nine years," he replied. "Can I get you some coffee or something else to drink?"

She shook her head and meandered over to his bedroom. He followed. He took the back of her head in his hand and started to kiss her, gently and with increasing passion. She slipped her hands under the hem of his shirt and pulled it off and they continued kissing. He leaned back to look at her and she noticed the scars on his body: two on his right shoulder, another on his abdomen, and smaller marks along his upper arms. When he noticed her looking, he turned around to lower the light, revealing the gashes across his back. She brushed her fingers along the deep marks. "I'm sorry," he said, turning to face her. "War wounds. A couple of gunshots. Some other stuff from when I was in the Gulf and later doing undercover work. I know it's gruesome."

"It's wonderful," she whispered.

"What?" he said.

"I'm sorry, I didn't mean it that way. It's just that I've never seen anyone whose outsides match my insides."

He looked at her sympathetically.

"I was abused when I was little. My grandfather and my uncle. It started when I was eight. No one can see my wounds, but they're there."

He stood still, looking at her.

"I'm so sorry. I've never shared that with any man I've been with in my entire life, and I just met you. That has to be the least sexy thing ever. I'll leave," she stammered, trying to walk past him.

He took her hand and pulled her back toward him. He cupped her face in his hands, gently caressed her cheeks, and kissed her. They made love with their eyes locked on to each other. Afterward, he held her in his arms and said, "That was so special. Spend the day with me tomorrow."

"Okay," she replied, and they fell asleep, their limbs entangled.

* * *

The next morning, Tess awoke to find a note on the pillow beside her that read, "Went to get breakfast. There's an extra toothbrush on the bathroom counter. Back soon."

She brushed her teeth, and by the time she was done, Jack had returned.

"Hey, sweetheart," he said, as if they had known each other for years. He pecked her on the cheek. "I didn't know what you like so I got bagels, muffins, and a fruit salad. Do you want coffee?"

"Yes, please. Black."

He poured two mugs of coffee and they sat down at the small table. "What kind of food do you like, anyway?" he asked.

"I'm a vegetarian. I don't believe in hurting living beings."

Jack looked down, a hint of shame on his face.

"Innocent beings," she said.

He smiled. "I guess that's why you're so tiny."

She started picking at the fruit salad. Jack noticed that she was moving it around with her fork, almost like she was counting. He looked at her quizzically.

"I'm weird with food. I don't eat that much. It's kind of a control thing." She paused, keeping her eyes on her breakfast. "I have problems."

He reached across the table and put his hand on hers. "That's okay. We all have problems. They make us human."

The pair spent the day together, talking, watching TV, and walking around Jack's neighborhood. They got Chinese takeout for dinner and made love twice more. Sunday morning, Tess realized she'd missed a dozen calls and text messages from Omar. She called him while Jack was making coffee.

"I promise, I'm fine. I'm sorry I worried you. I met someone. His name is Jack. He's special. . . . Well, if he is holding me hostage, don't pay the ransom. I want to stay. . . . I'll text you all about it. . . . Okay, love you too. Bye."

"He was worried about you?" Jack asked.

"He's been looking out for me for a long time. We talk every day, but I guess I was too preoccupied yesterday," she said, slipping her hands around his waist.

"Sounds like a good friend," Jack said.

"He's more than that; he's my family. He moved here a year ago and convinced me to leave LA so we could be in the same city. But enough about him. Right now, I'm only interested in you. Come here," she said, walking backward toward his bedroom. Just as he was about to touch her, she grabbed a pillow and walloped him.

"Oh, you're in trouble now," he said, darting for a pillow. They tumbled onto the bed, laughing.

They spent the rest of the day lounging around Jack's apartment, reading the Sunday newspaper, and sharing stories. That night before they went to sleep, Jack said, "I don't want the weekend to end. Do you have to work tomorrow?"

"Well, I do work for myself. Can you take the day off?"

"I once took two weeks off, but other than that, I've never taken a single day off in over twenty years. So yeah, I think I'm due for a personal day."

* * *

The next day, Tess and Jack went for a walk and ended up at a local park. They sat on a bench, huddled together in the chilly, late autumn weather. Suddenly, a little boy ran over and tugged at Tess's coat sleeve.

"Do you have superpowers?" he asked. "My dad says you do."

"Excuse me?" she said.

His father came running over. "I'm so sorry if he was bothering you, Ms. Lee."

"Not at all," she replied with a gracious smile.

"I'm a librarian. I want to thank you for everything you've done," he said.

"My pleasure," she replied. "Thank you for what *you* do."

The little boy tugged at her sleeve again. "Well? Do you have superpowers?"

His father laughed. Tess looked at the boy and lowered her voice conspiratorially. "I'll tell you a secret. Everyone has superpowers, they just don't know it."

"Even me?" he asked.

"Especially you," she replied.

Jack smiled.

The man took his son's hand. "I think we've bothered these people enough. Thank you again, Ms. Lee," he said, leading his son down the path.

Jack looked at Tess. "That was so sweet, what you said to that boy."

She leaned over and kissed him.

"What was the deal with his father? It seemed like he knew you."

"I did some volunteer work for the library a few months ago," she replied.

A few little girls came skipping past them, drawing their attention. Jack suddenly seemed far away. After a moment passed, Tess touched his hand, and he looked at her.

"It's starting to get cold. You want to go to a movie?" he asked.

"Sure."

After the movie, they went to a neighborhood Italian restaurant for dinner. The maître d' greeted Tess like an old friend. "Ms. Lee, such a pleasure. We have our best table for you."

"I guess you've been here before," Jack said as he pulled out her chair.

"Jack, listen to the music," she said.

"Sinatra—the best."

"Let's dance," she said.

He looked around. "I don't think they have dancing here."

"But I love to dance," she said.

He stood up, took her hands, and they danced by the table. "You know, I'm not much of a dancer, but I promise to dance to as many slow songs as you want."

"Maybe someday we'll have a special song," she said, nuzzling into his chest.

Later, when they got back to Jack's apartment, he led her to the couch with a slightly serious look. "I need to tell you something."

"What is it?" she asked.

"You've seen the scars on my body, but there's another side of it. Tess, I've done things—things that may be unimaginable to someone as sweet as you, things I had to do to protect innocent people." He proceeded to tell her every act of violence he had ever committed, his life laid bare at her feet. The list was long, the death count high.

When he finished, she said, "You did what you had to do for your job. I don't understand why you're telling me this."

"Because I'm in love with you. I'm completely madly in love with you and I've never felt that way about anyone. With the things I've done, I don't expect that you could ever feel that way about me, but I needed you to know who I am." He looked down.

She stroked his cheek. "Jack, I'm in love with you too. I spent our first night together memorizing your face: every line, edge, ridge, pore. I knew you were the best thing that would ever happen to me and I was afraid the memory would have to last a lifetime."

"Oh, baby, you've made me so happy. I feel like the luckiest man in the world."

"Jack, let's not worry about all of the details of our pasts. I want to leave the pain behind and just love each other now."

He smiled. "Okay, but maybe I should at least know how old you are and when your birthday is."

"Thirty-eight, and I never cared for holidays, including birthdays."

"Got it. Forty-two, and sweetheart, you're the only present I'll ever need."

She smiled.

"Let's go to bed," he said.

The next morning, Jack went to work and Tess went home. At the end of the day, they met at his apartment. "I have something for you," he said, holding out a velvet box. "I was passing an antique store and saw it in the window."

She opened the box to reveal a gold heart locket. She beamed and her eyes filled with tears. "Jack, it's the best present I've ever received," she said, putting it around her neck. "I'll wear it every day."

"You have my heart, Tess. My whole heart, forever."

"Promise me something. Don't ever buy me another present again. Nothing could ever be better than this."

"I'm hoping life is long. That's a lot of birthdays, holidays, Tuesdays," he said.

"Flowers. You can always get me flowers if you want to," she replied.

"Which ones are your favorite?"

"White hydrangeas. I never buy them for myself," she said.

They kissed, and then Jack got up and turned some music on. He reached for her hand. "Let's dance."

The second song that played was "All of Me." Two lines into the song, Jack said, "This is our song, I just know it is. Okay, baby?"

She nodded and rested her head on his firm chest.

They continued to work each day and spend each night together. Thursday night, Tess made eggplant parmesan, which she brought over to share with Jack. While they were eating, he said, "My friends and I go to this place called Shelby's Bar every Friday night. I told them all about you and they really want to meet you. Will you meet us there?"

"Of course," she said. "Tell me about them."

"Joe is in his mid-fifties. We've worked together for about fifteen years. He's a class act. Bobby is young, twenty-nine, and the nicest, most laid-back guy. He joined the Bureau three years ago, but I feel like I've known him forever. His girlfriend, Gina, is an elementary school art teacher. You'll like her."

"Sounds great. What do you think about bringing an overnight bag and staying the night at my place after we hang out with your friends? It's about time you see it. Omar and Clay are coming over for brunch on Saturday and I'm dying for you to meet each other. Will you?"

"Absolutely," he replied.

"Do you think it will seem strange to our friends, how deeply we feel about each other after such a short time?" she asked.

"I don't know. But no one can ever truly understand the depth of the darkness we've both survived, what we see in each other, and why we just want to love with our whole hearts. I can hardly explain it to myself. How could anyone else ever get it?"

"Jack, you know how people always talk about all the things they want to do or see in their lifetime? They don't even mention being happy because I suppose they think that's just a given."

"Yeah."

"Happiness has never been a given for me. I guess I pursued other things," she said.

"Me too," he replied.

"But I'm so happy now, with you."

"I love you so much, Tess."

"I love you too."

Reflection on *Shooting Stars*

The beginning of a novel is all about introducing the characters, establishing the setting, and highlighting themes to come. Fiction is character driven. I believe there is nothing more important in fiction than those who populate the story-worlds. Readers need to feel an emotional connection to characters to get into a story and care about what happens. Every time a character appears, it's an opportunity to show who they are. When developing a character, it's important to show who that person is from the outset. I attempted to do so in the preceding chapter. At the core, Jack is a protector. We see this from his initial encounter with Tess, which occurs when he intervenes on her behalf when another man at the bar is hassling her. Likewise, at the core, Tess is a kind person who truly sees others. This is evident from the outset when we hear her conversation with the bartender whom she just met, and then again, when she not only gives money to a homeless man, but takes his hand and looks into his eyes, and yet again at the park when we learn about her charitable work on behalf of libraries. Each moment is a chance to get to know the characters. Furthermore, we get to see the larger environment in which their story is playing out—from Tess's friend being pulled over for being Black and the homeless person they encounter—we immediately get a sense of the larger world of Washington, D.C., in which their story takes place.

Showing the relationships between characters, and what connects them, is also important, especially in a love story. Through their initial conversation in the bar and later at Jack's apartment when Tess sees his wounds and shares an intimate detail of her life, we learn that these characters become close because they've both experienced pain in their lives. Likewise they are both committed to sacrifice on behalf of others. This kind of intimate sharing bonds the pair, allowing deep trust between the two to quickly develop. They show us why they just want to love each other fiercely, leaving the darkness in their lives behind.

> When developing a character, remember that every time he, she, or they appear, it's a chance to show who they are. In the beginning, consider describing their physicality (e.g., gender, race, ethnicity, age, clothing, facial features, perceived attractiveness); what they do (e.g., profession, hobbies); their personality (e.g., shy, loud, funny, sarcastic, core values, ethics, how they make others feel), and most important their core motivation (e.g., what makes them tick, their essence or emotional center). Finally, name the character, bearing in mind that names carry all kinds of significance and may denote age, nationality, or religious background or give a character an "every person" quality. There are also alliteration considerations—how a name sounds, how it sounds in conjunction with other names, and if a nickname is going to be used.

Foreshadowing is an important literary tool in shaping a story—it gives readers a glimmer of what lies ahead, setting the stage. Foreshadowing was interwoven throughout the chapter. Often these are little things that don't necessarily register as significant, but then when more is revealed in later chapters, they make sense because of the ground that was laid earlier. For example, although we don't learn about the death of Jack's daughter, Gracie, until Chapter 3, in the opening chapter Jack mentions having once taken 2 weeks off. Later in the scene at the park, some girls go skipping by and Jack wants to leave, suggesting they go to the movies. Also during the park scene, we learn that Tess has done something to help libraries. Later at the restaurant, the host greets her by name, giving her the best table in the place. It's not until Chapter 2 that we learn Tess is one of the most famous authors in the world and has donated millions to libraries and other charitable causes. Finally, Jack gives Tess a gold heart locket proclaiming, "You have my heart, Tess. My whole heart, forever." The locket ultimately becomes pivotal during the climax of the book.

In these ways, Chapter 1 tries to cover a lot of ground by showing who the characters are, the larger environment they live in, how they bond, and foreshadowing events to come.

Twinkle

Twinkle follows Tess and Jack after 2 years of marriage. As they both heal from past trauma, their epic love, fostered by their ability to truly see one another, has brought them true happiness. However, when an anonymous threat is made against Tess's life, everything changes. Will they learn to lean on each other, or will they fall apart into the darkness? Once again, their friends are along for the ride. *Twinkle* is a novel about the nature of doubt, the struggle to feel worthy of love, the relationship of the small part to the greater whole, and the ways in which love from lovers, friends, or the art we experience can help us move from trauma to healing and redemption.

In the following chapter, Tess and Jack, along with a couple of their friends, attend a black-tie international arts and peace gala hosted by the president of the United States. Tess initially turned down the invitation. While she spent most of her adult life on the road, traveling around the world talking about her novels, the arts, and literacy, she hasn't attended events of that nature for the past 3 years. Jack has never seen her in that world—a world where everyone wants something from Tess Lee. However, when Jack is invited to the gala to represent the Bureau, Tess agrees to go, hoping to spend the night simply as "Tess Miller," the identity that grounds her and the way she wants her beloved Jack to see her. I selected this chapter because it is one of the longest in the series and provides an opportunity to talk about structuring long chapters and setting a stand-alone scene in a new environment. This chapter also shows how to weave minor characters into a narrative and mix humor with more serious subject matter.

Twinkle, Chapter 4

Jack was waiting for Tess in the living room when he received a message that the driver to the gala was outside. He knocked on their bedroom door to check on her, calling, "Hey, sweetheart, are you ready?" She opened the door. His jaw dropped and he put his hand on his heart. Tess was wearing an off-white gown with a full skirt and plunging neckline. The entire gown was adorned with crystals. "Almost ready, honey. I just have to put my necklace on," she said, picking up the gold heart locket she had worn every day since Jack gave it to her.

"Here, let me do that," he said. She swept back her dirty blonde hair, he kissed her neck, and fastened the chain.

She turned to him and said, "You are the most handsome man I've ever seen."

"You are so beautiful. You took my breath away," he said. He kissed her softly. "Shall we go?"

"Jack, I need to talk to you," she said anxiously.

"The driver's waiting. Can we talk in the car?"

"Sure."

As soon as they got in the car, Jack's phone rang. "It's the office. I just need to make sure everything's okay."

She nodded and watched as he answered the call.

He covered the receiver and said, "There's a situation and they need my input. I'll try to make it fast."

"It's fine," she replied, fidgeting.

As they pulled up to the gala, Jack was still on the phone. He noticed that Tess was nervously tapping her fingers on her leg, so he quickly wrapped up his conversation and hung up. "I'm sorry, sweetheart," he said. "You wanted to talk to me." He took her hand and realized she was shaking.

"We're here," the driver announced.

"We need a minute, please," Jack replied. He turned to Tess. "Sweetheart, what is it?"

"It's nothing. We should go in."

"Sweetheart, you're trembling. Tell me."

She turned to him and he caressed her face. "Jack, will you please do something for me without asking why?"

"Yes."

"When we leave this thing tonight, let's not talk, let's not say a single word. Let's just go home and make love and be us. No words. Please."

He leaned forward and gently pressed his lips to hers. "Okay."

"Thank you."

Jack told the driver they were ready but that he was going to get the doors himself. He stepped outside, opened Tess's door, and extended his hand. She took his arm and they walked up to the entrance. Photographers hollered, "Tess Lee, over here," and asked them to stop for a few pictures. They posed in the light of the flashbulbs, and then Jack said, "Shall we, Mrs. Miller?"

* * *

As soon as they were inside, they paused to take in their exquisite surroundings. "Wow, this place is really something," Jack said, admiring the ballroom that featured parquet floors and high ceilings dripping with crystal chandeliers.

Tess smiled.

Jack rubbed her fingers. "Look how pretty the tables are; they're overflowing with white flowers and candles, just like you love," he said. "And the orchestra is in full swing. I can't wait to spin you around the dance floor." She smiled. A waiter in a white jacket passed by, carrying flutes of champagne, sparkling water, and bite-size morsels, so Jack grabbed a sparkling water and handed it to Tess.

"Thank you, honey," she said, taking a sip.

People immediately noticed Tess and offered respectful smiles and nods. She did the same in return. Jack spotted Omar and Joe standing together.

"Butterfly, you look stunning," Omar said, hugging Tess.

"You look absolutely radiant," Joe said, leaning in to peck her on the cheek.

"Thank you. You both look as dashing as ever. Are Abdul and Layla here yet?"

Omar shook his head.

"Please tell me you finagled us seats together," Tess said.

"Uh, well, Butterfly, that's a funny story. Take a deep breath. The short version is that we're all sitting at the president's table."

"So, we're flying under the radar like I asked?" Tess joked, handing her glass to a passing waiter.

"Well, it seems that she's desperate to meet you and had planned to seat you and Jack at her table. When I spoke with the event coordinator to try to get us at the same table, I was informed that, and I quote, 'The president would be delighted to sit with Ms. Lee and her guests.' She wanted to speak with Abdul anyway. They've video conferenced. She's recently become quite interested in his counter-extremism initiative. So, this should be fun! Right, Butterfly?"

Tess rolled her eyes.

"Not bad, Tess. I guess Jack and I should stick with you. Seems you can teach us a few things," Joe said.

Tess feigned a smile and looked down. Jack grabbed her hand and whispered, "Are you okay?"

Before she could answer, a couple walked over. With a thick French accent, the woman said, "Tess Lee, this is a thrill. We're big fans of your work."

"Merci c'est très gentil," Tess replied.

"Ah, you speak French beautifully. It's wonderful that you're here. You do so much to support the arts," the woman said.

"Eh bien ce soir, je suis juste ici en tant que rendez-vous avec mon mari." She turned to Jack and said, "I was just telling them that tonight I'm here as your date."

"Bonsoir," the woman said.

"Bonsoir," Tess replied, and the couple walked away.

"You speak French?" Jack asked.

Before she could respond, she was again interrupted. "Tess Lee, I don't believe my eyes," a willowy man said in a British accent. "You are a vision," he continued, leaning in to kiss her on each cheek.

Tess recoiled and latched onto Jack's arm. "Hello, Oliver. Lovely to see you. This is my husband, Jack, our friend Joe, and I believe you know Omar."

They all exchanged polite greetings, and Oliver refocused on Tess. "You've turned down my last three invitations, or should I say, your assistant has. I can't even get a hold of you."

"I'm sorry, I've been busy. Remember when writers used to spend their time writing? Well, I'm trying to bring that back."

He chuckled. "You always were ahead of the curve. Come to London and we'll throw a bash in your honor. I won't take no for an answer."

"I'm afraid you'll have to. I really don't do events anymore."

"But you're here tonight, so there's hope," he said.

"Simply to dance with my husband," Tess said, intertwining her other arm around Jack's.

"I'm sure he won't mind if I cut in. Perhaps I'll convince you when we're on the dance floor. See you later, Tess. You are ravishing. Gentlemen," he said, before sauntering off.

Tess leaned over to Jack and whispered, "If you let him cut in, I'll divorce you."

Jack laughed.

"Who is that guy?" Joe asked.

"He's an insufferable little man. . . . " But before Tess could continue, Eliza Elkington tottered over, throwing her arms in the air. "Tess Lee, in the flesh. I've been wanting to do a profile on you for years. I talked my way into an invite to this thing as the date of some German cultural attaché. He's an absolute bore and I hope he doesn't think I'm going to sleep with him. Between us, the most he can hope for is a blow job, and I'd have to be plenty drunk for that."

Jack covered his mouth to mask his laughter.

"Anyway, it's all worth it now that I see you're here, Tess."

"Hi, Eliza. Nice to see you. This is my husband, Jack, and these are our friends. Eliza is the publisher for a women's magazine."

"Not a women's magazine, *the* women's magazine, darling. Well, you certainly married yourself an attractive man," she said, looking Jack up and down dramatically. "Maybe you'll take me for a ride around the dance floor," she said, batting her eyelashes.

Jack smiled politely. "Actually, I'm hoping to spend the night with my beautiful wife."

"Isn't he delicious, Tess?" Eliza gushed. She turned back to Jack. "Good luck keeping Tess to yourself. She's always in demand."

Tess looked down.

"Listen, I'm serious about the profile. We could make it a cover story. I'd love to spend a couple of days in Tess Lee's world, observing, interviewing. I know you're impossible to get, but I do love a challenge and I never take no for an answer."

Tess smirked.

"Promise me you'll think about it," Eliza said. "I'll get in touch with your assistant. Ta-ta!"

Tess smiled and Eliza sauntered off.

"She's enthusiastic," Jack said.

"That's one word for it," Tess replied.

They both laughed.

"You certainly are popular, Tess. It must be tiresome," Joe said.

Tess sighed.

"Butterfly, you didn't really think you could just be Tess Miller, did you? Still, that doesn't mean you can't enjoy yourself with your handsome, and dare I say, sought-after man. What will you do if he dances with Eliza?" Omar said, laughing.

"I'd pay good money to see that. It would be like dinner theater," Tess replied.

"If you let her cut in, I'll divorce you," Jack said.

"She'd eat you alive," Omar joked.

They all laughed.

Just then, the president walked into the room with her chief of staff. The group watched as she shook hands with several people before making a beeline over to them. "Tess Lee, this is an honor," she said, outstretching her arm.

"The honor is all mine, Madam President," Tess said, shaking her hand.

"I'm such a huge admirer of your writing and what you've done for the arts, women in business, libraries, I could go on and on. And you're a self-made woman to boot. I'm delighted we'll finally have a chance to chat. I've been trying to meet you for ages. You're harder to pin down than I am," she said with a laugh.

Tess blushed. "I believe you've met Jack and Joe, and this is my dear friend, Omar."

"Very nice to see you all," she replied. "Omar, I've seen your name on emails regarding Abdul's project. It's good to put a face to the name. My husband is out of the country on business, so Charles is accompanying me tonight. It never hurts to have your chief of staff at one of these things; it's so hard to remember everyone."

They all smiled.

"Madam President, Omar tells me that you've taken an interest in Abdul's counter-extremism project. That's wonderful," Tess said.

"Yes, it's a bold initiative. Several European countries have already stepped up to the plate. I wish I could raise more support for it in other parts of the world."

"Hmm, I see," Tess muttered. "Madam President, I hope I'm not overstepping, but may I ask you a question?"

"Please do," she replied.

"The G8 summit is only weeks away, and if one is to believe the news, terrorism will be at the top of the agenda. And you're hosting this gala, ostensibly for the arts and peace, with ambassadors from the Middle East as well as the G8 players in attendance. It hardly seems like a coincidence."

Everyone looked intently at Tess and the president.

The president smiled and glanced at Charles, who chuckled. She turned back to Tess. "I always knew you were brilliant. I told Charles on our way over here that I've just been dying to meet you. Yes, you're right. I was hoping to build some bridges for a broader counterterrorism initiative. The arts seemed like a, shall we say, gentle way to do that. It's been impossible to bring Japan to the table. I wanted to have the Japanese ambassador seated at our table, but was told that just getting him to say hello to Abdul would be an impossible feat. It goes both ways. They're being quite stubborn. It's turned an otherwise jovial occasion into something a bit more stressful."

Tess smiled. "I see. Who's representing Japan at the gala this evening?"

"Ambassador Kaito Harada," she replied. "He's here with his wife and a few of his aides."

Tess scanned the room. Omar winked at her and they covertly exchanged conspiratorial smiles. Just then, Abdul and Layla arrived, walking straight over. Everyone exchanged warm greetings.

"Madam President, it's an honor to finally meet you in person. Thank you for your support," Abdul said.

"Likewise," she replied.

He turned to Tess and embraced her lovingly.

"I'm so happy to see you, Abdul," Tess said. "Layla, you look stunning."

Layla smiled.

"I've missed you, my light. We are very glad to see you," Abdul said. "Although I must confess, I was surprised when Omar informed us you would be here. I thought you'd given up this life for the simpler pleasures you enjoy."

Tess smiled. "I'm making an exception tonight. Jack was invited, and you know how I love an orchestra."

"I see," he replied.

"Well, shall we find our table?" the president asked. "Tess, you're sitting next to me. We have so much to talk about."

Tess looked at Jack, who smiled and whispered, "You're so damn smart." He squeezed her hand and they headed to the table.

* * *

Tess was seated between the president and Jack, across from Abdul, their table in the center of the room and directly perpendicular to the band. Tess and Jack engaged in their own conversation about how pretty the flowers were and how divine the orchestra sounded, staring lovingly at each other, Jack rubbing Tess's arm. Waiters came over, introduced themselves, and promptly served drinks. The eclectic group made small talk.

"Layla, how was your trip?" Tess asked.

"Very good, thank you. We stopped in Paris on the way," she replied.

Tess smiled. "Abdul, were you looking at venues for the Paris events? Omar told me a little about it."

He nodded. "We have summits scheduled in Paris, Cannes, Milan, Venice, Frankfurt, London, Cambridge, Toronto, Vancouver, Abu Dhabi, Dubai, and several in the United States. It's become a much larger project than we could have imagined. The participating countries have all donated generously, each underwriting all of the expenses for the events."

"Omar and Tess mentioned something about counter-extremism events," Joe said. "What exactly are you planning?"

"We have designed a program that uses the arts to counter extremism and promote peace. We're hosting weeklong summits in cities across the world over the next five years. The participants will include leaders, policymakers, religious figures, artists, military personnel, scholars, and citizens from various walks of life. Each group will be carefully curated. We've been laying the groundwork for many years."

"That's remarkable," Joe said.

"It truly is," the president said.

Abdul smiled. "It has been the effort of many." He turned his attention toward Jack. "You must know that Tess inspired this project, yes?"

Jack looked at Tess with an inquisitive expression and placed his hand on her thigh. "I had no idea, but I can't say I'm surprised."

Abdul smiled. "Yes, I first had the idea when I read her fourth novel, *The Island,* years ago."

"Of course," the president said. "That's one of my favorite books."

Joe smiled. "I should have realized. I love that book."

Abdul continued, "But her influence did not end there. We spoke about it and she suggested how I might make it a reality. She contacted her network and worked her magic to line up the resources and key players."

Tess shook her head. "Abdul flatters me. I really didn't do anything."

Abdul laughed. "I see some things never change."

"You know what hasn't changed? How much I love to dance, and as I recall, you are quite light on your feet. If Layla wouldn't mind. . . . " Tess said.

"He would love to dance with you," Layla said.

Abdul smiled. "With Jack's permission."

Tess rubbed Jack's hand and he said, "Of course."

Abdul extended his hand and Tess rose to meet him. The group watched as they made their way to the far side of the dance floor. Tess stopped right in front of Kaito Harada's table. She looked at him and bowed her head almost imperceptibly. When the song ended, Kaito Harada stood up and approached Tess and Abdul. They exchanged words and the two men shook hands. "Well, I'll be damned," Charles said. "Madam President, are you watching this?"

"I sure am."

Tess began dancing with Ambassador Harada as Abdul strolled back to the table.

"I see Tess knows Kaito Harada," the president said.

"Tess knows everyone; she is very loved," Abdul replied. "She helped

Mr. Harada with an art education initiative in Japan years ago, and she is always his personal guest when she does book tours in Tokyo."

"I told you Tess would know just about everyone here," Omar said to Jack.

They all watched as Tess and Kaito danced, engrossed in conversation. When the song ended, someone on Kaito's staff approached to speak with him. Tess headed back to the table. Jack stood up and pulled her seat out for her. "I'm sorry, baby," she whispered.

He lifted her hand to his lips, kissed it, and winked at her, and they both sat down.

She slowly took a sip of her sparkling water and placed the glass back on the table with great care, then turned to Jack and said, "Have you ever been to Japan?"

"No," he replied.

"Tokyo is one of my favorite cities in the world and Kyoto is enchanting, especially during fall foliage and the spring bloom. I would love to go there with you."

"I would love that."

She squeezed his hand and turned to Abdul. "Abdul, the president mentioned you have been in negotiations to bring Japan on board. Wouldn't it be wonderful to have them participate in your project?"

The president and Charles shot each other a look. Everyone eagerly waited at the edge of their seats for the response.

Abdul smiled. "Yes. We tried, but we could not get them to commit. There are other politics at work that they refused to table. The negotiations went poorly and we were deadlocked. I was disappointed."

"Kaito and I just spoke. I explained how important the program is and outlined all the reasons that it would be in their best interest to join. He agreed," she replied. "They are willing to commit to cooperative events in Tokyo, Kyoto, and Osaka, following your model."

Everyone's eyes widened.

"That's wonderful news, Tess, but there must be a price to pay. We offered many things during the negotiations and it was never enough. What must we surrender?" Abdul asked.

"Nothing," she said. "There's just a small gesture. It's nothing, really."

Abdul raised his eyebrows skeptically.

"All you have to do is get up and walk over to him. You must be the one to extend yourself."

Abdul looked down and let out a heavy sigh. "You know what you are asking."

"I know what it signifies to Kaito, but I also know the kind of man you are." She lowered her voice. "It's meaningless. Remember who you are. See this place for what it is. This is only the realm of the 1 percent. Nothing that happens here matters. There is only darkness and light, and love is the bridge between them. Your program is love. Think of the 99 percent to which you've devoted your life. Do you know what I see when I look around this room? Many men who have abandoned everything that once mattered to them for the chatter, for the false trappings of the elite. It's heartbreaking," she said, a tear falling down her cheek. "This gesture," she paused, crinkled her nose, and whispered, "it's meaningless."

Everyone sat with bated breath, the president's eyes glued to Abdul.

"Thank you for your counsel, Tess," Abdul said.

Tess smiled faintly and lowered her chin. "Of course."

A moment passed as Abdul thought quietly. "I would like to take your advice, but how do I know that Mr. Harada will follow through if I make the journey to him?"

"It would be my pleasure to personally escort you and Layla."

Abdul turned to the president. "Madam President, I hope you will excuse us for a moment."

"Certainly," she replied.

Abdul and Layla stood up. Tess whispered to Jack, "I'll be right back." She walked over to Abdul and linked her arm with his. The three approached Kaito, who stood and extended his hand as soon as they arrived. Jack, Joe, Omar, the president, and Charles watched with their mouths hanging open.

"Holy mother of God," the president said. "If I hadn't seen it with my own eyes. . . . " She turned to Jack. "Do you have any idea what your wife has just done? She's extraordinary."

Jack smiled humbly. "Yes, she is."

A few minutes later, Tess excused herself and turned back toward her table. En route, several people stopped her to chat. Jack couldn't take his eyes off her, a slight smiled etched onto his face. Eventually, she made it back to the group. "I'm sorry, baby," she whispered as he pulled her seat out.

"Don't be," he said.

When she sat down, everyone looked at her, their mouths agape.

"It's done. Japan is in. They're making plans, and it turns out Layla and Kaito's wife have quite a bit in common. Perhaps they'll all become friends," she said.

"Well done, Butterfly," Omar said, raising his glass.

"It was nothing," she replied. "Although I don't understand why you didn't just ask me to make a call from the outset."

"Abdul insisted we leave you out of it," Omar replied.

"That's curious," she replied.

"Tess, I consider myself a master negotiator but I've never seen anything quite like that. You certainly live up to the legendary tales I've heard. How on earth did you manage that, let alone in the ten minutes we've been here?" the president asked.

"Kaito is quite old fashioned when it comes to gender roles. I'm sure you're used to dealing with men like that, Madam President."

Everyone laughed.

"I knew that if he saw me, he'd feel obligated to ask me to dance. That was my chance to have them shake hands and exchange pleasantries as a courtesy to me. When I was dancing with Kaito, I had the perfect opportunity to bring up Abdul's project and explain why I thought it was in his country's best interest to participate. He values my opinion. He's not a man who is willing to give something for nothing, but I explained the need for equity for the program to work. Of course, he demanded a gesture, a show of power. Kaito operates from a hierarchical notion of respect, hence forcing Abdul to make the journey to him."

"What about Abdul?" Joe asked. "What was all of that about the 1 percent?"

"Abdul cares more about peace than politics. He wanted to say yes, but I had to give him a way to live with it. Although it was merely symbolic, it was still a concession. Abdul and I used to study different religious texts and mysticism when we were touring the Middle East. In some regions, our lives were constantly under threat and we were literally trying to take the guns from people's hands and replace them with paint brushes, pens, and books. Abdul needed spiritual guidance. We read quite a bit about Kabbalistic thinking. One thing we could both agree on was the notion that everything we see in this realm—these flowers, those candles, the designer gowns, and the necks dripping with diamonds—it's only 1 percent of what there is in the universe. Our souls exist in the 99 percent, so we must not become distracted by the frills of this superficial, material realm."

"You're brilliant, Tess," Joe remarked.

She shook her head. "You're very kind."

"He's right. You led him exactly where you wanted him to go," Charles said.

She looked at him sharply. "No, I would never do that. I led him exactly where *he* wanted to go. It has nothing to do with me." She turned to the president. "Now I hope you can enjoy your evening without the added stress you mentioned earlier."

"Is that why you did all that?" she asked in disbelief.

"Jack and Joe have devoted their lives to fighting terrorism and this program will diminish the need for that work. It will make the world a little safer. It was also good for both Abdul and Kaito and those they represent, and you, after all, are our host. Sometimes things are in everyone's best interest, if we can only recognize that," Tess replied.

"You are a wise woman," the president said.

Tess blushed. "Madam President, I hope you don't find me rude, but my husband promised me a night of dancing, and so far, it's all been with other men."

They all laughed. "Certainly, please enjoy yourselves," the president replied.

"That's my cue," Jack said. He rose, took Tess's hand, and led her to the dance floor. He placed his hand on the small of her back, pulled her close, and said, "You are breathtaking and I love you beyond words."

She smiled. "Let's just dance."

* * *

Tess and Jack danced for ages. Several men asked to cut in, but Jack politely said, "I'm sorry, not tonight." Finally, they rejoined their group, holding hands and smiling at each other like two people in on a private joke. As they sat down, the first course was served.

"Thank you, Jerome," Tess said to the waiter. "This looks nice," she said to Jack, admiring the red and golden beet salad.

"I made the pumpkin recipe you gave me, Tess," Layla said. "It was delicious and so aromatic."

"Oh, that's one of my favorites. I'm glad you liked it. I can't take credit; I got the recipe from a friend in Afghanistan."

"Yeah, that friend just happens to be the president of the country," Omar said.

"No, it's his brother. He's a lovely man and a wonderful cook. I know his brother is a bit more, um, complex," Tess said.

Joe laughed. "That's diplomatic."

"You don't have normal friends," Omar said.

"You're right. I have you," she quipped.

Omar rolled his eyes playfully. He then turned to Charles and Joe and engaged them in conversation.

The president focused on Tess. "Do you like to cook?"

"Yes."

"That's one thing I miss. I used to love cooking, and especially baking. I found it so relaxing, a way to decompress and sort through my thoughts," the president said.

"I suppose you don't have time anymore," Tess said.

She shook her head.

"What do you do for pleasure?" Tess asked.

The president sighed. "The two things I loved were reading and baking. I still manage to read. I never miss a Tess Lee novel."

Tess smiled. "I can only imagine the demands on your time and that you feel obligated to use it for the benefit of others, but perhaps it's also important to do things that are restorative. I can recall countless reports of former male presidents playing golf, tennis, fishing, or even surfing. I'm sure you have an incredible kitchen at the White House. I hope you can give yourself permission to use it."

The president smiled. "Thank you, Tess. I actually miss having girlfriends to sit around the kitchen with, make a pot of coffee, and bake cookies. Of course, we never talked about bake sales, more like foreign policy and funding for the arts, but that was the way we did it. The people I know in Washington aren't really those kinds of friends."

"I suspect it's hard to have those types of relationships once you're in your position. Everyone wants something from you, even just to be near you," Tess said.

"Indeed. I imagine that's something we share in common. No one warns you about the loneliness, do they? You can be surrounded by admirers and yet feel totally isolated. I guess we should be grateful to be too busy to think about it," the president replied.

Tess smiled. "Oh, I don't know. I thought that for a long time. But at some point, perhaps it's good to pause and make sure that we are powering the rocket and not just holding on for dear life."

The president let out a huff. "Yes, perhaps. Now tell me, what you love most is writing, yes?"

"Since I was a girl."

"Your novels are sublime. You can capture the balance of pain and hope in our lives like no one else. When I need courage or inspiration, I read your work."

"That's very kind," Tess said.

"I've noticed that you use the same dedication in each of your books, since your debut novel. You always write 'to everyone, everywhere.' That's lovely."

Tess smiled.

"What's your creative process like?" the president asked.

"It's different every time. That's why I'm still in love with writing. Sometimes, I get a complete idea, like a movie unfolding before me. Other times, I just have a character that I can see and hear. Sometimes, I know the last line and I write my way to it. It never happens the same way twice."

The conversation continued and soon the salad plates were cleared. The band resumed playing.

Joe approached Tess and said, "I know Jack wants you all to himself, but I would love to steal a dance with you."

"There's no need to steal what I'll happily give you," she said, rising and taking his hand.

Omar turned to Jack. "I'm going to stretch my legs. Want to head to the bar for a real drink?"

"Sounds like a plan."

Once at the bar, Omar threw back a shot of vodka.

"You okay?" Jack asked. "You don't usually drink very much."

"Can I ask you something?" Omar replied.

"Sure."

"If a woman hit on you, no, if a woman propositioned you, would you tell Tess?"

"Listen, it's just a matter of how much you trust Clay. For what it's worth, I really don't think he's the type of person to cheat."

"But what would you do if a woman came on to you?" Omar pressed.

"I'd shut it down in a way that was crystal clear. Would I tell Tess? If there was something funny about it that I thought we could laugh at, sure. Otherwise, probably not. I wouldn't see any reason and there'd be no point upsetting her."

"Thanks. I know you're right, it's just my insecurity talking. Clay is ... Oh, shit. Incoming," Omar said as a man made a beeline toward them. "Thank God I did that shot. This guy makes my ears bleed. Jack, whatever he says, please stay calm."

Jack looked at him for an explanation but there was no time.

"Omar, well I'll be damned. Great to see you," the man slurred in a southern drawl.

"Hi, Dick. What brings you here?" Omar replied.

"Hang on, I need a refill." He turned to the bartender. "Top it off. Bourbon."

"You sure you need another?" Omar asked as Dick grabbed his drink so forcefully it sloshed about in the glass.

"Ah hell, I need something to get through this night. You know the company donates a shitload to the arts for the write-off."

"How touching," Omar muttered.

Dick took a swill of his drink. "Bernard Bentley told me you got him mixed up in some international project. You should have come to me."

"And why is that?" Omar asked.

"My bank account's bigger," he said, erupting in laughter. He composed himself and continued, "Don't worry about me; I got a girl back at my hotel for later, the kinda girl who does what you say. But I'll tell you, man to man, I'd drop her in a flash if you could get me a night with Tess. Hell, Tess can have me for as long as she wants, and I don't say that about most women, course most women ain't worth as much as I am. That Tess, she's such a tiny little thing, but I'd love to bend her over and . . ."

"And let me just stop you right there and introduce you to Tess's husband, Jack Miller."

"Well no shit, Tess tied the knot."

"Uh, yes she did. Jack is a federal agent. Basically, he's spent the last couple of decades killing people, professionally."

Dick burst into laughter. He stuck his hand out, "Dick Clayton. Good to meet you. Hope there's no bad blood. I've had a hard-on for Tess for years. Didn't know she got married."

Jack carefully placed his glass on the bar, stared daggers at the tactless buffoon, and softly said, "Don't speak that way about my wife or any woman ever again." He turned to Omar and said, "I'm going back to the table."

"Coming right along with you," Omar said. "Good night, Dick. Have fun with your hooker or whatever. Try to avoid getting arrested."

On their way back to the table, Omar said, "I'm very impressed that you didn't pummel him."

"It wasn't easy, but I didn't want to cause a scene. Who was that asshole?"

"Oil tycoon. Tess only knows him because he buys his way into events like this. She uses her extensive network to raise money for the arts and literacy, including from his company, always putting the cause above all else. She can't stand him."

When they got back to the table, Jack sat down. He put his hand on Tess's back, leaned over, and said, "I just met Dick Clayton."

"I'm so sorry for you. Which did you find more repellent: his arrogance or his misogyny?"

He laughed.

"At least he's well named. If ever there was a dick," she said.

He kissed her cheek and said, "Sweetheart, I need to feel you in my arms. Would you like to dance?" Before she could respond, a man approached the table.

"Excuse me, Madam President. I hope I'm not intruding," he said.

"Not at all," she replied.

He turned to Tess. "Are you Tess Lee?"

"Yes," she replied.

He smiled brightly. "I am so humbled we can finally meet in person. I am Ebo, Pireeni's colleague. We have exchanged many emails."

Tess jumped up and hugged him like an old friend. "I'm so glad to meet you. The work you do is incredible. Ebo, this is my husband, Jack." They shook hands, and she introduced him to the group. "Ebo works with several orphanages in Ethiopia. He created an arts and literacy program for the children there."

The president stood up and shook his hand. "That's very commendable."

Everyone echoed the sentiments.

Ebo turned to Tess. "If I may, I wanted to show you photographs of what you have made possible. You must see the children with their books and the art projects they have created. It has been life changing for them." He slid his phone out of his pocket and started scrolling through pictures. Tess started to tear as she watched the photos whiz by. "They're amazing," she sniffled.

"I do not wish to disturb your evening any further," Ebo said, pocketing his phone. "I'm grateful for the chance to thank you in person."

"Thank you for all that you do," Tess said, clasping his hands.

Ebo said good-bye and walked away. "Sweetheart, are you okay?" Jack asked.

"I just need a minute," she said. "Please excuse me," she said to the group and dashed out of the ballroom.

"Jack, what was that about? He thanked her," the president asked.

"I don't know," he replied. He sat down and turned to Omar.

"Tess funded the entire program, every penny. It was meant to be anonymous. She doesn't like attention for these things, so you probably shouldn't say anything when she gets back."

"Wow," Charles muttered.

"I'll say," Joe mumbled.

"Is Tess all right?" the president asked.

"Tess does much good in the world, but she does not like to dwell on it. When she is forced to contemplate what she has done, she does not think about the children she helped, only the ones she cannot help. She feels the suffering of others deeply. It has made her a gifted writer, a perceptive analyst of the human condition, one who knows that the shadow side of pain is hope, as you suggested, but there is a grave personal cost," Abdul said.

Jack stood up. "Please excuse me." He walked out into the lobby and waited outside the restroom. When Tess emerged and saw him, she smiled and softly said, "Hey."

"Hi, sweetheart. May I have this dance?"

She nodded, a tear falling from her eye.

"Oh hey, come here," he said, enfolding her in his arms.

* * *

"That was delicious," the president said, as the waiter cleared the dinner plates.

"Thank you, Jerome," Tess said as her plate was removed.

"Tess, you hardly ate a thing. How was the eggplant?" the president asked.

"It was fabulous, thank you. I'm just not very hungry."

Jack took her hand under the table, brushing his fingers against hers.

"How long have you been vegetarian?"

"Since I moved away from home when I was nearly eighteen. I just can't bear to hurt living beings."

The president smiled. "That's interesting, given what Jack does for a living. Certainly not that he wants to hurt anyone, but the nature of his work."

"Sometimes the world requires us to do things we'd prefer not to do, so we sacrifice some part of ourselves for the greater good and we try to find a way to live with it. That's something I understand," Tess replied.

"You understand too well," Abdul said. "I hope someday you understand less."

Jack brushed the side of Tess's face. She leaned into it and looked into his warm, blue eyes. "I love you," he mouthed.

"I love you," she mouthed in return.

The president was about to say something when the waiter interrupted. "Excuse me, ma'am," he said to Tess. "A gentleman asked me to deliver this to you." He handed her a note. She read it and said, "Thank you, Jerome. Where is he?"

The waiter pointed across the room. She peered over. The man held up his glass and smiled. She raised her glass and smiled in return. "What is it?" Jack asked. She handed him the note, which read:

Rumor has it your husband won't let anyone dance with you. I wanted to say hello. M.

"Who's M?" Jack asked.

"Mikhail Petrov, Russian minister for the arts. He's a special friend. You'd like him; he tells the dirtiest jokes I've ever heard."

"Is he here with his goons?" Omar asked, craning his neck to look.

"He never goes anywhere without personal security," Tess replied.

"Oh, and I see he brought Svetlana. That explains why he's bored and passing you notes like in grade school," Omar said.

"She's not that bad," Tess replied.

"Butterfly, have you ever tried having a conversation with her? She couldn't find Russia on a map."

Everyone laughed.

"Perhaps she has other charms," Tess said. "I like Mikhail."

"I never trust a man who travels with personal security and whatever Svetlana is," Omar rebuffed.

Everyone snickered.

"But this does explain a strange conversation I had earlier," Omar said. "Serge approached me and asked about you and Jack."

"Well, that's irksome. What did he want to know?" Tess asked.

"Just how serious you two are," Omar replied. "Relax, I told him you're madly in love and that it's going to last forever. Now I realize he was inquiring for Mikhail. Seems he's still in love with you."

"Oh please, you're ridiculous," Tess replied, as she reached for Jack's hand under the table.

"Tess, you've certainly led an extraordinary life. I can only imagine the stories you could tell," the president said.

"Actually, I think I've only recently gotten to the good part," she replied, rubbing her fingers against Jack's. Jack smiled as they looked at each other out of the corners of their eyes.

"I've met Mikhail a couple of times, but I can't say I have a good sense of what kind of man he is," the president continued.

"He cares about the arts and culture, but corruption surrounds him. Personally, I've always gotten on very well with him. He can talk about philosophy and poetry for hours, he's hilariously funny, and he drinks like a fish," Tess said.

"I'll give you that, Butterfly. I don't know how he was still standing after doing all those gruesome cherry vodka shots in that bizarre little bar. It really did look like a brothel."

Tess giggled. "It did. That's the night I tried smoking a cigar. God, that was dreadful."

"Butterfly, I told you not to inhale."

She shrugged. "It was fun. You must admit, Mikhail knows how to entertain."

"Plus, he did nearly kill a man for you. I guess if you're willing to forget how bloody scary that was, one could almost view it as gallant," Omar said.

"Oh hush, he did no such thing," Tess protested.

"I'm telling you, if that man walked out of there alive, he was probably missing a few fingers," Omar said.

Tess shook her head. "You're overly dramatic."

"What happened?" Jack asked.

"We were in a private room in a Moscow bar with a smattering of diplomats, ambassadors for the arts, and so on. You know, Tess's usual, utterly surreal group of friends."

"They weren't friends," Tess argued. "They were acquaintances."

"Some man from Mikhail's outer circle had too much to drink and tried to get a little too friendly with Tess. Mikhail, inebriated and blinded by his feelings for her, almost killed him. First, he nearly broke his hand, or quite possibly did. Then, he threatened him. It was all in Russian, so I don't know exactly what he said, but that man was scared for his life. Then, Mikhail had his goons remove him. I'm telling you, he never made it home, certainly not in one piece."

"I'll admit that things got a little heated, but everyone settled down and it was fine. I really think they just asked that man to leave. Let's not get distracted with stories about Mikhail's drunken escapades. More importantly, did you and Abdul try to get Russia on board with your project?" Tess asked.

"That's even funnier than watching Svetlana try to read a map," Omar replied.

Joe and Charles cracked up.

"It isn't possible. They would never work with us," Abdul said.

"Really?" Tess muttered. She turned her attention to the president. "Madam President, now that Russia is back at the G8 table, wouldn't it be wonderful if they signed on to Abdul's project? Then you'd have all the players working cooperatively on something. That could only mean positive things for diplomacy in general."

"I'm afraid I agree with Abdul. It's not possible. Even if we could get them interested, which is beyond a long shot, I can only imagine what they'd try to strong-arm us out of in return."

"Abdul, do you remember when we were touring the Middle East and we approached that checkpoint crawling with armed men? Our security insisted they would make us turn back," Tess said.

Abdul laughed. "You truly have not changed. Yes, of course I remember. You are right. One should never give up before they have tried."

"Honestly, I think you're all right and that they'll say no, but isn't it a conversation worth having?" Tess asked.

"What are you thinking?" Charles asked.

"I don't know. Mikhail will speak with me, but I'd need to brainstorm what to say. You're all quite right—they have no interest in working with any of you, no offense."

Everyone laughed. "You are candid, Tess. A woman after my own heart," the president said.

Tess smiled. "There would have to be a new angle, a motivation we haven't considered yet. The biggest problem is that he doesn't have autonomy. He won't make a single move without first getting clearance from above. He has the Russian president on speed dial. Mikhail is smart; he understands the implications of using his budget and influence to do anything international. It's just after ten here, which means that it's just after six in the morning in Moscow. That's workable, at least."

"Butterfly, he won't do this just because of his feelings for you."

Tess rolled her eyes. "Of course not, but he will listen in earnest to what I have to say."

"I admire your determination, but it really can't be done," the president said.

"You're probably right, but it seems worth a few minutes of our time to be certain," Tess replied. She turned to Jack. "What do you think Russia truly wants at this moment? It's not peace, it's not cooperation with the West, and it's certainly not freedom or funding for the arts."

"Power," he said. "They want power."

"Yes. And power is different from capital. Wealth is flashy, but power...."

"Power conceals itself," Jack said.

"Exactly, you're brilliant," she said, leaning over to kiss him. "Honey, I need to speak with you privately," she said softly. He leaned closer and she whispered, "Mikhail and I had a very brief thing. It didn't mean anything to me, and it was ages ago. I think of him as a friend. I can only have this conversation with him if I go alone, but if it makes you uncomfortable, I won't. Would you mind?"

"Of course not. I trust you implicitly," he replied, stroking her cheek with the back of his hand.

She pulled a pen out of her purse and wrote something on the back of Mikhail's note.

"What did you write?" Jack asked. She handed him the note, which read:

I have a proposal for you. Meet me at the bar. Leave your thugs behind. Tess.

Jack smiled.

"Butterfly, before you do this, please answer one question I've always been curious about. You're right that Mikhail is smart and knows how to have a good time, qualities one should never undervalue. But I know how discerning you are; there's something else you like about him. What is it?" Omar asked.

She smiled. "Remember when he hopped on the jet and traveled the Baltic States with us?"

"How could I forget? That book tour became nothing but bars and night clubs. I had dark circles under my eyes for weeks. It was fabulous."

Tess giggled. "When we stopped in that little gelato shop in Riga, he ordered a scoop of vanilla. When you take all of this away, that's who he really is. And that is why we understand each other. He will hear what I have to say, even if we have to do the dance for the benefit of others."

Omar chuckled. "I understand."

Tess put her hand up to signal for a waiter. "Jerome, please deliver this to that man." She watched Mikhail as he read the note. He laughed, held up his glass, and smiled.

"Ah, he laughed. He's in a good mood," Tess muttered.

Mikhail got up and meandered over to the bar.

"Even if this is futile, I really must say hello to him anyway. Please excuse me," she said. As soon as Tess left, Jack turned to Omar. "Is he really in love with her?"

"Since the moment they met. You'll see. But he also respects the hell out of her."

Jack watched as she glided over to the bar, looking like a princess, her gown sparkling under the light of the chandeliers. Mikhail picked her up and dramatically spun her around in the air, paying no mind to the dozens of inquisitive eyes. Then, he put her down and kissed her on both cheeks. They leaned against the bar and began talking.

"I don't understand," the president said. "What was all of that about vanilla ice cream?"

"That's Tess-speak for 'he keeps things simple.' That's why she likes him. It's her favorite quality; it goes hand in hand with honesty," Omar replied.

Jack smiled.

"Brace yourself, Jack. This could take a while. I once watched the two of them debate a minute aspect of Nietzsche's work for hours. I was like, 'Bloody hell, I'll just Google it,' but they preferred to spar," Omar said, sipping his wine.

"Who won the debate?" Jack asked.

"Tess did, and I'm not really sure how. Mikhail and the others were all hell-bent on their perspective. It got absurdly heated. Russians take this stuff so seriously. I could see that Tess had enough of it. She leaned over and whispered something to him. He turned bright red, laughed, and declared that Tess was right."

Jack laughed.

"Your wife really is something," the president said.

"Yes ma'am, she is," Jack replied.

"If anyone can do this, it's Tess. I have seen her accomplish the impossible before," Abdul said. "She has rare talents. It's interesting because the American media portrays her as quite complex, but I have always thought the opposite. She has a decidedly simple, uncluttered perspective about the world and people. Do you agree, Jack?"

"Yes, I do. You know, on the day of our wedding, Tess told me you are one of the only people who really understands her."

"She is extremely dear to me. Tess has two very special gifts. Her first gift is her ability to witness people. I could point out that she is the only person at our table to call our waiter by his name this evening. She sees everyone."

They all looked down, huffed, and smiled.

"Her second remarkable gift is story. People cannot understand how she is so talented in both the arts and in business, but it is just those two gifts. In tandem, they explain both her literary and business prowess. She truly sees people and knows how to reach them. Then, of course, is the purity of her singular motivation: love. People know that when they speak to Tess, there is no other agenda. She sees only darkness and light, and she doesn't care about politics or power. She never lies. There is no manipulation. Whatever she is saying to him right now, I promise you she believes it. There are no games. This is why people trust her so unreservedly. With all due respect, Madam President, it is the reason why no politician could broker this deal, but why if anyone can, it is Tess."

They watched in stunned silence. "Madam President, are you seeing this?" Charles asked. "He just pulled out his cell phone. He's making a call."

"Unbelievable," Joe muttered.

They tried not to stare as Mikhail spoke on the phone for several minutes, becoming increasingly animated. When he hung up, he and Tess continued talking. She leaned over, whispered something to him, and he nearly fell over laughing. Then, he took her hand and led her to the dance floor.

"Well, this is going to make Svetlana's head explode," Omar joked. "She's always been hugely jealous of Tess. Everyone knows he's hung up on her."

Jack let out an audible huff. "I can see that, but I can hardly blame him."

They all watched as the two whirled around the dance floor. Mikhail said something to Tess and she laughed hysterically. At one point, she turned to Jack and winked. He smiled. When the song ended, they walked over to the table. Everyone stood up to greet them.

"Madam President, it's a pleasure to see you again," Mikhail said.

"Likewise," she replied, shaking his hand.

"Omar, nice to see you," Mikhail said.

"It's been too long, Mikhail. We were just talking about that wild little bar you took us to in Moscow."

Mikhail smirked.

Tess introduced everyone else. "Abdul," she said, "since you and Mikhail will be working together, I wanted you to have a chance to meet." After chatting for a few minutes, Mikhail said, "I better get back."

"Yes, it seems your date is waiting for you," Tess replied, glancing over at Svetlana, who looked like she was breathing fire.

"Oh, please," Mikhail said. "I'm going to the bar."

Tess laughed.

Mikhail turned to Jack. "Many men would cut off their hands to be with your wife."

"Or someone else's hand," Omar muttered. Tess shot him a look of admonishment and Joe muffled his laughter.

Mikhail continued unfazed. "You are a lucky man, Jack. Congratulations." He said good night to the group and walked off.

Tess blushed. Jack brushed the hair away from her eyes and whispered, "He's right about one thing: I am the luckiest man in the world."

They all sat down. Tess coolly took a sip of her sparkling water and finally said, "As you heard, they're in."

The president's eyes were like saucers. "I'm speechless. What have we given them?"

"Nothing. It certainly wasn't my place to give them anything," Tess replied. She looked at Abdul. "They'll host events in Moscow and St. Petersburg. It's not perfect; there will be a fair amount of censorship regarding the participant list and content, but that was inevitable. So, expect that they'll be modifying the program quite a bit."

Abdul grinned from ear to ear. "How can I thank you?"

Tess shrugged. "It was nothing. Abdul, you know the types of connections I have. Why didn't you and Omar use my name or ask for my help? I would do anything for you and your cause."

His expression turned solemn. "You are always generous, but I know that what you seek is not in this room. I did not want to drag you back into the 1 percent. Tess, my light, please hear these words as I heard yours earlier: you deserve that which you seek. Do not feel that you must sacrifice any part of yourself. You have already given so much."

Tess looked down. Jack caressed her hand.

"I don't understand, Tess. How did you make this happen without major concessions in return?" Joe asked.

"I kept it simple. I agreed with Jack that they want power. But of course, they don't want to be viewed as the brutes that much of the world thinks they are. This program, if viewed as a public relations strategy, solves a deeply rooted image problem. Mikhail took my point and was able to convey it up the chain of command. In that light, we are offering them an opportunity. Mikhail is pragmatic. Besides, I did him a favor years ago and I think he was pleased to repay it."

"Well, I don't know what to say. Tess, you've been my favorite author for so long and I was hoping to impress you tonight, but it's been just the opposite," the president said.

"Madam President, you are already impressive. You needn't try, it's self-evident."

"Good. Then I'm hoping you might come and visit me one day. Perhaps we can make a pot of coffee, bake some cookies, and discuss foreign policy or funding for the arts. I would love to be your friend," the president said.

"I would be honored," Tess said.

"See? No normal friends," Omar said with a chuckle.

They all laughed.

Dessert was served, meringues filled with lemon curd and dripping in berry sauce.

The president stood and said, "I've had such a wonderful time with all of you that I've neglected to make the rounds. There are many people I must say hello to. Please excuse me."

Jack put his hand on the small of Tess's back. "Sweetheart, would you like to dance?"

She nodded. "Desperately."

On the dance floor, Jack said, "So, you took him on your jet? Should I be jealous that he picked you up and twirled you around?"

"He just did that to piss off Svetlana. You should never be jealous of anyone or anything. You are the most incredible man in this or any other room, and as I told him, you are my everything."

"I know, I just wanted to hear you say it."

She looked at him intently.

"He's in love with you."

"Oh please, you've been spending too much time with Omar," she rebuffed.

"I saw the way he looked at you. It's undeniable."

"That's it, you and Omar can no longer play together."

He laughed. "Okay, we can talk about someone else who loves you: the president."

Tess smiled dimly but her expression turned forlorn. "Honey, I'm sorry if tonight wasn't what you hoped for. I feel terrible. I wanted to help Abdul, and all the people here know me, and it's impossible to . . ."

He leaned in and kissed her. "You have nothing to apologize for. Let's go home, Mrs. Miller. I have a promise to keep."

Reflection on *Twinkle*

A chapter that occurs in a new and distinct location—in this case, the gala—needs to be set up. The chapter begins before Tess and Jack arrive at the event, allowing me to describe the setting through their eyes, which helps establish the place, people, and mood. It includes the introduction of a plethora of minor and supporting characters. These characters are woven in, one by one, from the outset to help paint a picture of the people who populate this space. Dialogue was used to quickly show who each character is through their manner of speaking (e.g., accent, tone), their demeanor, their conversation, and their attitude toward others.

Beyond the set-up, there are two "writerly" issues involved in developing this lengthy chapter: delivering the content and the structure.

Content-wise, this chapter had three primary goals: building the start of a relationship between the president and Tess, further developing Tess's character, and delivering thematic content. It's clear how the president and Tess befriended one another, so I'll elaborate on my approach to developing Tess's character and advancing the book's themes.

Part of the job of this chapter was to show who Tess is: smart, respected, kind, compassionate. Readers need to see her through the eyes of other characters, so in addition to showing her interactions and conversations, storytelling was employed. This is a writing strategy, a device. At various points other characters who know Tess well—Abdul and Omar—talk about her to the others. We learn about Tess's generosity and her struggle to balance darkness and light through her friends. When Tess is off chatting with Mikhail Petrov, we learn that her favorite quality is "keeping it simple." This tidbit, revealed during a conversation in which Tess is not present, speaks volumes not only about her as a person, but also about her deep connection to Jack. Even in the smallest moments, writing may convey multiple things at once.

Thematically, *Twinkle* explores the relationship of the small part to the greater whole and picks up on the theme of darkness and light in *Shooting Stars*. These themes are interwoven throughout the chapter in ways that move the story forward. For example, when Tess brokers the deal between Abdul and Kaito, she discusses the 1% and 99% as it's understood in Kabbalistic thinking. During the same conversation she says, "There is only darkness and light, and love is the bridge between them." These themes were repeated when Tess excuses herself from the table, overcome with emotion after meeting Ebo, and Abdul explains the toll these encounters take on her. Again these themes are revisited after Tess brokers a deal with Mikhail and asks Abdul why he didn't come to her for help, and he responds that he did not want to drag her back into the world of the 1%.

Structuring a long chapter is challenging. Pacing, organization, and signposting need to be considered. Beginning with pacing, it's important to think about how to keep readers' interest while parceling out a lot of information. This chapter was divided into scenes in order to isolate characters and the many topics covered. In doing so, I strove to create balance between humorous and more serious moments. The organization of scenes is vital, and contrast or juxtaposition are useful tools in this respect. For example, different versions of masculinity are portrayed throughout the chapter. In one scene Dick Clayton's humorous but deeply misogynist conversation at the bar is contrasted immediately by Ebo's tender conversation in which he embodies generosity and compassion. These interactions were carefully organized. Last, when writing a long chapter, signposting, or returning to earlier events, is a useful way to bring a sense of closure. As one example, early in the chapter Omar jokes that Tess doesn't have normal friends. This joke is reinforced near the end of the chapter when the president asks Tess to be her friend. Looping back in this way helps summarize content and bring a sense of conclusion to an isolated scene.

Constellations

Constellations follows Tess and Jack after 3 years of marriage as they navigate the meaning of love and family over a series of holidays. What will happen to their blissful union when Jack's childhood family resurfaces? When Tess and Jack visit the Millers for Christmas, how will insecurity, a sense of missed opportunities, and the need for redemption test their relationship? When a terrible accident threatens everything in an instant, will they learn the true meaning of unconditional love? Once again, their loved ones are part of the story, but this time they include the Miller clan. *Constellations* is a novel about families—those into which we're born and those we create—the human desire to belong and feel connected, the true and multilayered nature of intimacy, and the power of love to heal and redeem.

The following selection is the epilogue from *Constellations*. At the climax of the novel Tess was hit by a car on Christmas Eve, after shoving a 4-year-old girl named Genevieve out of the way, saving her life. Tess's accident reminded Jack of the death of his daughter, Gracie, at the age of 4. The accident serves as a catalyst for Jack to reconnect with his childhood family, who finally learn he had shut them out of his life because of the dangerous nature of his work as a counterterrorism field agent. The epilogue takes place the day after Easter, which Tess, Jack, Omar, and his husband, Clay, spent at the Millers' house in Pennsylvania. I selected this chapter as an example of an epilogue. It also includes an excerpt from one of Tess's novels, which I wanted to share, particularly because it evokes the central metaphor used in the book as a means of summing up, so it's an opportunity to highlight metaphor and closure. Honestly, I just love this epilogue so much, I had to include it.

Constellations Epilogue, "The Next Day"

Mary drove Jack and Tess to the library an hour before the scheduled reading and discovered that the streets were lined with cars a mile in every direction. When they arrived at the library, they were stunned to see a mob waiting outside and several police cars coordinating crowd control.

"Thank goodness I can park in one of the reserved spots," Mary said. "You two wait here while I see what's going on."

When Mary returned to the car, she said, "It seems that thousands of people have shown up for your reading, dear. They've come from all over. The police won't allow everyone in because we've far exceeded capacity. They say it's already standing room only. Thankfully, I had them put signs on the chairs in the first two rows, reserving them for our family and the Pattersons."

They all got out of the car. Jack took Tess's hand and they walked slowly through the crowd to the main entrance. People were taking pictures of Tess on their cell phones as she smiled and said "hello" and "thank you for coming." Many were holding copies of her books, and she promised to come outside and sign them after her reading. Mary rushed Tess through the crowd inside to a back room where she could wait. On the way, she noticed people with piles of her books on their laps, some with overflowing tote bags. Jack waited with Tess until fifteen minutes before the reading, and then left to join his family in the audience.

After he left, Tess cracked the door open to sneak a look at the audience. Jack, the Miller clan, Omar, and Clay were seated in the front row. The Pattersons, including Genevieve, were seated behind them. She returned to the back room and texted Omar: *Please come see me.*

"Butterfly beckons. I'll be back in a flash," he said to Clay and Jack.

A few minutes later, Omar rushed over to Jack. "I need to speak with you privately."

Jack followed him to a quiet spot in the back of the library near Tess's waiting spot. "What's up?"

"Slight hiccup. Tess is nervous. Nervous is an understatement, really. She's completely freaking out."

"Seriously? Tess never gets nervous."

"I know. She's spoken in front of presidents, prime ministers, and rock stars; she's been in arenas all over the world in front of thousands, and done countless talks guarded by men holding machine guns, not to mention a slew of high-profile television appearances. The one thing my Butterfly has never gotten is butterflies. Suddenly, at this modest library in the middle of Pennsylvania, she's practically hyperventilating. Everything I say seems to make it worse."

"What did you say?" Jack asked.

"Well, a pep talk is new territory for us, so I tried reminding her that she's Tess Fucking Lee. She said, 'Oh my God,' and started pacing in a circle. Then, I tried reminding her she's Tess Miller. She threw me out of the room. In all the years we've known each other, I've never seen her nervous."

"I have, once: the day we announced that we were getting married. She cared so much about what you would think and was a wreck. This is because we're all here."

Omar smiled. "Of course. Can you help? If she hasn't escaped through the window, she's in there," he said, pointing to the back room.

"I'm on it. Go sit with everyone," Jack said.

Omar nodded.

Jack knocked on the door.

"Yeah," Tess muttered.

He opened the door and found Tess leaning against the wall, her head between her knees, trying to catch her breath. He walked over and rubbed her back. "Sweetheart, what's wrong?"

"I think I'm having a panic attack. I'm not really sure because I don't know what they feel like, but I sort of think it must feel like this."

"Calm down. Deep breaths," he said. "It's okay."

She raised her head and looked at him. "I feel like I'm going to pass out and my heart is racing."

"You've done a million of these things. What's going on? Talk to me, sweetheart."

"It's just..."

"What, baby?"

"I never had a family there before."

He smiled and put his hand on her face. "Yes you have. You've had Omar and you've had me."

"This is different," she said softly.

"Come here," he said, embracing her. He wrapped his arms tightly around her, encircling her in his protection and love. "They're your family. They love you. There's nothing to worry about. Just stay here in my arms until you're ready."

After a couple of minutes, Tess pulled away.

"Do you feel better?" Jack asked.

She nodded. "You're my rock. You always make me feel better."

"They love you and you can count on it. It's real, sweetheart. Just lean into it. Be you. That's all anyone wants."

"Kiss me, Jack."

He kissed her gently. "I love you with my whole heart, forever."

She took a slow, deep breath. "I love you too. Okay, I'm ready now."

Jack walked Tess to the doorway, where she was asked to wait to be introduced. He kissed her again, smiled, and returned to his seat. He nodded at Omar, letting him know everything was okay.

Mary approached the podium and tapped the microphone to make sure it was working. "This is a very special treat for our community and for my family. Tess Lee is one of the most celebrated authors in the world. Her novels have inspired hundreds of millions of people, showing them that there is a path through their pain, light on the other side, and infinite possibilities for love, hope, and redemption. I couldn't be more excited to introduce one of America's most prolific, honored, and beloved authors, and a woman I personally love very much, my daughter-in-law, Tess Lee."

Tess emerged to a massive standing ovation, her family in the front row. She placed her silver pen on the podium, with the words Tess Miller oriented to face her. She smiled at Jack and began, reading selections from fan favorites *Candy Floss, Blue Moon,* and *Ray of Light.*

"Before we get to the book signing, I wanted to do something I've never done before. I hope you'll indulge me as I read an excerpt from the unpublished novel I'm currently working on."

Everyone clapped vigorously.

"It's called *Holiday Homes,* and it's about family, something I've been thinking about a lot lately. Really, it explores loss, missed opportunities, and the human need for connection that we all share. I started writing it when I was here last, and it's dedicated to my family seated right there in the front row," she said gesturing and smiling. Jack smiled at her and she began reading.

"She walked down the no-name street in a no-name town in small town America, wondering where she belonged. As the cold

December air hit her face, she looked at each house, imagining the different kinds of families, each warm and toasty inside. Suddenly, a scream. She turned to see a little girl, headlights upon her. Racing over, she shoved the girl to safety. In the flash of light, she saw the face of the daughter that couldn't be saved; someone else's daughter would have to do, a different family to remain whole. After the car slammed into her body, she lay on the cold concrete, the noise around her fading, a feeling of peacefulness washing through her. It's a clear night, she thought, staring at the dark sky lit up with stars. I hope the little girl is okay, the little girl saved from the headlights, and the other one who could not be saved, still shining brightly like a star that died long before its light reached us.

"She saw Orion, the hunter. Is the hunter seeking something she doesn't yet have, or is she seeking something already within, she wondered. When the hunter finds what she longs for, will she return home? What treasures will she bring the others from her travels? As she lay on the frozen ground, she decided that Orion was her favorite constellation. She laughed, thinking about how everything is connected after all. There are no accidents. Constellations are like families, just random groups of stars, near each other by chance, but they recall something familiar to us, so we see a pattern in the randomness. The universe was made up of stars and people who found themselves clumped together by chance, because someone walked into a bar one night, wandered onto a football field one day, birthed a child one morning, or fell in love with someone in an instant. And yet, there's something so familiar, so clear it feels like it couldn't be any other way. And so, we cling to the connections.

"She heard voices telling her, 'Stay with us.' She tried to tune out the noise. There were still questions to answer. Why do we look at the stars? Is it to imagine other worlds or to connect us to our own, like the very stardust of which we are made? Where do I belong? If I return to stardust, will I be a part of a constellation? Will he look up in the night sky and see me, a pattern in the randomness? The voices became louder. 'Stay with us,' they beckoned. Okay, she thought. My stardust shall remain here for now, with him, with them, with the imperfectly perfect, impossibly possible family of which I'm a part, by choice or by glorious happenstance."

Reflection on *Constellations*

Final words always have a big job. This is where you pull everything together; it's what readers are left with.

Each novel in the serial ends with Tess speaking, but in this case, I chose to end with Tess's writing so that ultimately she weaves together the threads of the novel, taking readers to the journey's conclusion and showing her character's evolution. The epilogue taps into the human desire to belong—the desire for connection and intimacy, a sense of "family," and Tess's quest for something real and steady after a life spent globe-trotting, surrounded by others, but feeling alone. Furthermore, the metaphor of constellations was introduced earlier in the novel and now is returned to at the end, demonstrating how this kind of literary device can be used to build meaning. Here constellations are a metaphor for families, and as it is central to the story, this metaphor became the title.

> A quick formatting tip: if you're creating an excerpt from a book, newspaper story, diary, letter, text message, or other document, I recommend using a different font to clearly distinguish the different voices and sources from which the characters are reading.

Words always matter to writers, but there are moments in a novel where words matter even more. Sometimes we need something beautiful. Sometimes we need to feel all the feelings. The last three paragraphs of the epilogue strive to bring the book's themes together through the beauty of language and deep wells of emotions readers may feel by this point. Furthermore, the patterns Tess sees and the questions she asks leave readers something to ponder in their own lives.

Supernova

Now blissfully married for 4 years, one catastrophic event is going to change everything and push Tess and Jack's relationship to the brink. Can Tess move through this new trauma? Will Jack's need for vengeance destroy their relationship? When trust is violated, can there be forgiveness? In order to find their way through to the end, Tess and Jack will need to go back to the beginning. *Supernova* is a novel about walking through our past traumas, moving from darkness to light, and the ways in which love from lovers, friends, or the art we experience heals us and helps us learn to forgive ourselves and others.

Supernova is the heaviest of the novels in this serial. It delves deep into the wounds created by past trauma, and many difficult subjects are covered. In the climax, while socializing with her friends at a salsa bar, Tess sees one of the men who repeatedly raped her when she was a child. Jack sends Tess home with a friend, and then follows her abuser to his home where he assaults and threatens him. When Tess learns what Jack has done, she's so traumatized at the thought of his violence, that she flees to Omar and Clay's apartment. The following passage is a brief excerpt from Chapter 8, in which after quarreling with Omar, Tess goes outside for some air.

Supernova, **Excerpt from Chapter 8**

Tess stood up and opened her handbag. She retrieved a pack of cigarettes and a book of matches. "I'm going outside for some air," she said.

Ten minutes later, she was sitting on the stoop puffing away on her second cigarette when Omar came outside. "May I join you?" he asked.

She shrugged.

He sat down beside her. "When did you start smoking again?"

"I bought a pack last night. Don't give me a hard time."

"I won't." They sat in silence for a couple of minutes. Eventually, Omar said, "Tess, you're right and I'm sorry. I know you're going through a dreadful time right now and I'll support you any way you choose. I do respect you beyond measure. I only want to help. All I know is how much you love Jack and how happy he makes you."

Tess took a drag on her cigarette and stomped it out. "I don't know if I can ever be with him again after what he did. I've never felt so lost and heartbroken in my life, not for a moment, nothing like this pain."

"Butterfly, I'm so sorry," he said, rubbing her back.

"When I couldn't sleep last night, I watched something on TV about supernovas, which is basically when massive stars explode. They say a supernova is so luminous that it's like an entire galaxy, but then there's nothing, just a black hole. Maybe that's like me and Jack. I always felt like we burned so brightly, but maybe now after this explosion, there won't be anything left to salvage. We just won't exist anymore."

"You know, I saw part of that special too." He leaned back on his hands and looked up at the sky. "What I remember is that the shock wave created by a supernova can cause the formation of new stars. Maybe that's what it will be like for you and Jack. Yes, you're going through something hugely dark right now, but maybe from this experience you'll create new light."

Reflection on *Supernova*

I selected this excerpt as an illustration of how to initially weave metaphor into the story, while continuing to move the plot forward, and indeed foreshadowing what is coming. Themes of darkness and light had already been peppered throughout the narrative, and in this scene the supernova metaphor is introduced. When using a device of this nature, it's important to be clear and precise with your language. I tried to do this with this short conversation. Here I hope you can see how metaphor is used to illuminate relationships, build tonal content, punctuate themes, and foreshadow possible outcomes. The metaphor is returned to at the end of the novel.

I also used this brief extract as an example of titling a project. As with *Constellations*, the central metaphor also provided this book's title. Titles can be simple, but they ought to be meaningful. Ultimately, the meaning of a title should be revealed.

North Star

North Star follows Tess and Jack after 5 years of marriage. As they both heal from past trauma, their epic love, fostered by their ability to truly see one another, has brought them true happiness. However, when life's challenges arise and two significant forces from Jack's past resurface, everything they've learned about unconditional love is put to the test. Will they finally live their lives happily ever after? Will they finally learn to let go of the darkness and live in color? In addition to new characters, their long-standing friends play supporting roles. *North Star* is a novel about commitment and letting go, loss and gain, and the ways in which love in all its forms can help us move from trauma to healing and redemption.

North Star is arguably the lightest novel in the series, offering my version of a happily-ever-after. I wanted to represent some of that lightness. Tonal balance is important. I compare it to a soufflé. The humorous scenes are the light and airy part. When you dive deeper, you find something rich and decadent. It's created out of a balance of airiness and richness.

The following chapter takes place at Shelby's Bar, where Tess and Jack regularly meet their friends for fun nights out. Although each novel deals with trauma, they also each include many lighthearted scenes written with humor, and so I wanted to share one such example. These lighter chapters are a break from the drama, yet are still central to moving the plot forward. I've especially used these chapters as a chance for Omar and Tess to share stories from their past, showing their long and deep friendship, as well as the grandness and in some cases surrealness of Tess's extraordinary life. To give some background, to her surprise, the previous evening Tess had an award named in her honor, which was presented by her friend, the president of the United States.

North Star, Chapter 4

Friday night, Tess and Jack arrived at Shelby's Bar to find Omar, Bobby, Gina, Joe, and Luciana already seated at their regular table by the dance floor. As the Millers approached, everyone started clapping.

"You guys," Tess said, blushing as she and Jack sat down.

"We got you drinks," Bobby said. "We have to toast this."

"Congratulations, Tess," Joe said, raising his beer bottle.

Jack draped his arm around Tess. They all raised their drinks and said, "Congratulations!"

"Thanks," Tess said, sipping her sparkling water.

"Tess, I know you aren't comfortable with the attention you receive for your work, but this is well-deserved. We're thrilled for you," Joe said.

"What you've done has changed the landscape of art. Even those of us who work in the visual arts are deeply inspired. Your work is a shining example of the best of what the arts and artists can do," Luciana said.

"You're all very sweet," Tess said.

"Were you surprised?" Gina asked.

"Very. Honestly, I thought we were there to celebrate my friend Abdul's work. I had no idea. I'm especially surprised Omar didn't tell me. He and I are supposed to have an understanding," she said, picking up a pretzel and flinging it at him.

"I must confess, Butterfly, I was terrified of a repeat of Edinburgh. I told Clay all about it. He wanted to be here tonight to tell you what a nervous wreck I've been, but the hospital called."

"What happened in Edinburgh?" Bobby asked.

"Well, I *thought* what happened was that Omar promised never to surprise me with an award again. Apparently, my memory fails me," Tess said.

Omar laughed. "Indeed, Butterfly. To be fair, I was under presidential orders this time, so I didn't have much of a choice. Besides, I didn't think Jack would let you arrive a loopy, slobbering mess."

"I wasn't slobbering," Tess protested.

"Uh, yes you were. If it's any consolation, Butterfly, they probably just all thought you were tipsy. Eccentric writer and all."

She picked up another pretzel and lobbed it at him. "I still can't believe you let that happen."

"Okay, I can tell this is a good story. Spill," Bobby said.

"Butterfly, shall I tell them, or do you want to do the honors?"

"Since I barely remember the evening, it's all you."

Omar laughed. "It was over fifteen years ago. Tess had been traveling around Europe, promoting one of her books and giving talks about the humanities and arts. I met her in the UK at the end of the tour. We spent a few nights in London, during which Tess was on a nonstop schedule of book signings, public talks, and press junkets, not to mention social obligations every night. Then we flew to Scotland, where Tess was supposed to attend an arts and literacy soiree. Little did she know, she was to receive a major award that evening. The entire event was in her honor and she had no idea. When it was time to leave for the gala, I knocked on the door to her hotel suite. She didn't answer. I called, no answer. Luckily, I had a key to her room, so I let myself in. Tess was fast asleep. It took me eons to wake her up. When I did, I learned she had decided to skip the gala and had taken not one, but *two* sleeping pills, probably on an empty stomach. I could barely keep her conscious long enough to even ascertain that much."

"Let me stop you right there. I hadn't slept properly for weeks. I was exhausted. As far as I knew, it was just another gala. I took two pills, hoping it would knock me out for the night."

"That it did," Omar said, bursting into laughter.

"It isn't funny. The whole thing was mortifying," Tess said.

"Indeed it was," he said, trying to compose himself.

"What did you do?" Joe asked.

"Well, I managed to get her into a seated position. I told her that the gala was in her honor, that she was receiving an award, and would be expected to make a speech. Her eyes whirled as she tried to process what I was saying. She kept saying, 'What?' really slowly," he said, bursting into laughter again.

"It isn't funny," Tess said, chucking another pretzel at him.

"Anyway, I convinced her she had to go to this thing, no way around it. Then I called room service and had them rush up a large pot of coffee. FYI, it's a myth that coffee will help in that kind of situation. All it did was make her need to go to the bathroom every five seconds."

They all cracked up.

"So anyway, Tess had canceled her hair stylist and makeup artist, but she assured me she could do it herself. I should have paid more attention to the fact that she was slurring her words and couldn't quite walk straight."

Tess shook her head. "It isn't funny."

"What happened?" Bobby asked.

"She managed to do her hair and get into her gown, but there was a slight hiccup with her makeup. She must have confused her lipliner and her eyeliner, because she emerged from the bathroom with hot pink lines around her eyes and a dark brown outline around her mouth, like some sort of psychotic clown," he said, dissolving into hysterics.

They all started laughing so hard they were falling out of their chairs.

"Oh my God, I can't breathe," Jack said, taking a swig of his beer.

Tess looked ready to throw the entire basket of pretzels at Omar. "It was all your fault," she said.

"Admittedly, Butterfly, I can see that now. But hindsight, as they say."

"You didn't let her go like that, did you?" Gina asked.

"Of course not, but it was a delicate situation. She was hardly in top form and I didn't want to let on that she looked ridiculous. I told her she needed a slight touch-up. I sat her down in the bathroom and fixed her face as best I could. I mean, bloody hell, what do I know about makeup? At least she didn't look like a circus performer by the time we left. I did my best to keep her awake on the car ride over, not an easy task. The event was in this massive, gothic castle. We arrived horribly late, and the hosts rushed out to greet us." He stopped to laugh. "I'm sorry, Butterfly, but it really was hysterical."

"I hate you," she quipped.

"Love you too. Anyway, they all had incredibly thick Scottish accents. I could barely understand them myself, and Tess was completely out of it. I knew she couldn't understand a bloody word they were saying. Not a word. She just kept smiling vacantly at everyone. Then they grabbed her hand and pulled her inside. She turned to look helplessly back at me, like she had no clue what was going on."

"I didn't," she said.

"Well, it all worked out in the end. I stood just offstage with her as they presented her award, you know, trying to keep her from toppling over or drooling. But I have to give you credit, Butterfly—when you got on stage, you were stunningly coherent."

"Yeah, well I guess I had the Tess Lee thing down pat. Apparently, I can even do it in my sleep."

Omar smiled. "After that, a few men whirled her around the dance floor like a rag doll until I was able to make our excuses and get us out of there."

"Yes, and when I woke up the next morning...."

"Uh, when you woke up the next *afternoon*," Omar interjected.

"Yes, well, I only remembered bits and pieces of the night."

"Probably best that way," Omar said, laughing.

"No doubt. But I do remember making you promise to never put me in that position again. You swore you'd never keep something like that from me. Now I see what that promise was worth."

"Oh, come on, Butterfly. It all worked out. If it helps, I really have been a nervous wreck hoping we wouldn't somehow have some surreal repeat."

"I can't believe you didn't tell me about this, Omar," Jack said.

"Trust me, I was trying to spare you from the anxiety, and I didn't want to jinx anything," Omar replied, taking a swig of his beer.

"So, thankfully last night went a lot smoother. Tess, tell us: how does it feel to have this award named after you? It's quite a legacy," Joe said.

She took a deep breath and said, "Honestly, with the award and the launch of my foundation, I feel like I might be saying good-bye to a piece of Tess Lee, like this theater tour is a farewell in some way. Maybe life will become simpler, quieter."

Jack squeezed her and gently kissed the side of her head.

"I'm quite certain that's enough award talk for a lifetime. Right now, Jack and I are just excited about adopting a dog tomorrow. What's going on with everyone else?"

"Well, Bobby and I have some big news. We're expanding our family too. I'm pregnant! Rob is going to have a little brother," Gina said.

"Oh, wow! Congratulations! That's wonderful news," Tess said.

"Congratulations!" everyone said.

"And Tess, like you, there's a part of my old life I'll be saying good-bye to," Bobby said. "Joe's the only one who knows; I asked him to keep it quiet. I'll be changing positions at the Bureau, moving out of the field to a desk job."

"As someone who's been there, that's a big move," Jack said.

"Gina doesn't like me doing a job that requires me to carry a gun and wear a bulletproof vest. Now with a second kid on the way, I need to put them first."

Gina smiled and patted his arm.

"Congratulations. It's great news. You'll find your footing in your new role in no time," Jack said.

"If it doesn't work out, I have a buddy with a construction company and he promised to hire me," Bobby said.

Just then, a slow song came on the jukebox. Jack leaned over and whispered, "Would you like to dance, Mrs. Miller?"

Tess smiled and nodded.

Jack took her hand and led her to the dance floor. He held her close and they started to sway.

"That's some pretty major news," Tess said.

"Yeah, they always wanted a big family. It's great."

"No, I mean Bobby taking a desk job, or possibly even leaving the Bureau."

"I can understand why better than anyone. It's not a job that mixes well with family. He's prioritizing Gina and the kids."

"And what do you think about that? Do you think he'll regret it?"

"It's just a question of commitment. He's making his family his number one priority. It's the right call."

She gazed into his eyes. "Jack . . . " she whispered.

"Yeah, baby?"

"I love you, that's all."

He smiled, leaned forward, and kissed her lightly. "I love you too, sweetheart."

Reflection on *North Star*

This chapter is an example of one contained real-time scene completely driven by dialogue. Friendship and humor are an integral part of this series. Scenes at Shelby's Bar are one constant where friendships are celebrated with lots of laughs.

The close friendship between Tess and Omar is the second central relationship in the series. They are soul mates with a long history of loving and supporting one another. Added to that, the friendship group that formed when Tess and Jack fell in love is also an important part of their story. These scenes at Shelby's Bar, which typically center on storytelling and humor, are an opportunity to showcase these friendships. Humor and storytelling—as seen in the discussion of the "Edinburgh incident"—are critical tools for adding a backstory, which further develops the characters and their relationships while also adding lightness to the novels. Given Tess's extraordinary or as Omar would say "surreal" life, my imagination ran free coming up with past experiences the two of them shared.

> Flashbacks are a common device for providing a backstory. However, if you want to write a narrative that unfolds in real time, you can use storytelling to achieve this same end. Characters share stories from their past in conversation with others. This is a specific way of employing dialogue that unfolds in real time, while allowing for background details.

These scenes are never ornamental, but also move the plot forward, even subtly so. In *North Star*, Tess and Jack are contemplating taking a big leap in their lives, but Tess secretly harbors the fear that their life together may not be enough for Jack. In this scene, she tries to feel this out with him when they're on the dance floor talking about Bobby leaving his job. As is often the case in the series, one character may try to work things out in their own life by relating to what's going on with other characters.

I've learned over the years that the more fun I have writing something, the more fun readers tend to have. When something makes you giggle or laugh, it's likely to have the same effect on others. As much fun as the characters have in these bar scenes, I had just as much fun writing them and I hope that joy comes through to readers.

Reflection on *Celestial Bodies: The Tess Lee and Jack Miller Novels*

Penning this serial was unlike any other experience of my life—the way the story came to me, how quickly it happened, and the way I approached the writing. Truly, of everything I've written so far, these books are nearest and dearest to me. Writing them was an immersive creative experience unlike anything else, and the resulting novels hold my hands more than anything I've ever written.

One day *Shooting Stars* came to me in a burst, which was quite different from the way my other novels have materialized. Usually, I stew on an idea for a while, and then spend a year or two drafting a manuscript.

Shooting Stars came to me quickly, and I wrote the entire first draft in about 10 days. I barely slept, I didn't respond to emails, and if anyone spoke to me, I'm sure I didn't hear a word they said. I was completely immersed, more than I'd been with anything before. It was magical.

I spent every waking moment of every day and night mentally in this story's world. It was an engaging, emotional, and cathartic experience. The writing process was completely different from that of my previous novels. In the past I had always drafted a rough outline and then written in chronological order. I viewed *Shooting Stars* as a compilation of scenes, and that's how I wrote it—completely out of order. The last chapter in the book was the first one I wrote, then I skipped around in the middle, and I finished by writing the first chapter. In fact, because there was no outline, I had no idea how many chapters there would be so I saved each one with names like "cake scene" or "cereal scene," confident that in the end I would be able to string the scenes together. The structure of this novel is completely organic; there was no formula. By abandoning everything that had worked for me in the past, I was able to achieve something new. *Shooting Stars* could not have been written any other way. The process pushed me creatively and made me a better writer. How was I able to do this in 10 days? It was possible because of the discipline and skills I developed over many years. When the moment of inspiration and opportunity presented itself, I was ready to serve as a scribe and allow the story to come through my filter. Although I had experienced magical moments of discovery when writing previous novels, those moments were just fleeting. With *Shooting Stars*, the entire process was magical—one of cocreation with a source of inspiration that somehow came to me as if it had been waiting all along.

Differing from previous works, *Shooting Stars* takes place entirely in real time. I didn't utilize some of the literary devices I've used in the past. There's no interior monologue, nor are there any flashbacks. These choices were made so readers could experience these characters as they experience each other: together and in real time through their interactions and dialogue. Instead of relying on flashbacks, I use storytelling as a way of providing a backstory, in which

> As you develop your writing style, allow yourself to evolve as an author. Just because a certain process has worked for you in the past doesn't mean it will always work or that you shouldn't try new things. Try writing in different structures. Try writing chronologically. Try writing out of order. Try new things for new projects.

characters share stories from their past with others. In terms of other literary tools, I also used foreshadowing, dropping subtle clues throughout. Themes were interwoven in numerous ways, including through dialogue, symbolism, and metaphor. For example, the theme of darkness and light shows up through dialogue, but also through clothing, photography, the sky at different times of day, and by other means. Let's take clothing, which may seem innocuous at first glance, but was consciously chosen throughout. Tess and Jack only wear black, white, and gray, representing darkness and light and their attempt to balance the two. The only time the colors change is when they are in Hawaii, their special place, where they wear bright colors (and ultimately in *North Star* where they learn to live in color).

After I finished drafting *Shooting Stars*, I fell into a deep depression for 24 hours. This was the best writing experience of my life, and I felt strongly that it was also the best thing I'd ever created. Finishing it was devastating. Would I ever feel that way again? My heart also ached for the characters that had become so near and dear to me. Waking up without racing into their world left me with a profound sense of loss. I missed them. While I always experience some measure of sadness when finishing a novel and saying good-bye to the characters that have occupied my days, this time it was worse. I knew more about them and loved them more than I was able to share in one book. We only had 10 days together. It wasn't enough.

Standing out on my balcony looking up at the sky, suddenly I realized there was much more to explore about love through these characters. Again, in a burst, *Twinkle* came to me. I immediately started writing. This time, I knew it wasn't merely a sequel, it was a part of a serial. I drafted *Twinkle* in about 12 days in the same manner as *Shooting Stars* by writing scenes out of order. The next books followed, each drafted in between 10 and 20 days. Novelists often know much more backstory about their characters than comes through in a book. There's so much I knew when writing *Shooting Stars* that didn't emerge until later books— for example, Jack's family, the Millers, who don't show up until *Constellations*, or his best friend, Jones, who doesn't appear until *North Star*. These novels were all written in the same manner: out of order as scenes in real-time, using dialogue, interaction, storytelling, foreshadowing, metaphor, and symbolism, and without imposing any structure.

Here I'll pause to note that while these novels were drafted quickly, they were each revised dozens of times, in addition to receiving peer feedback and professional copy editing. Magic came in the first draft, and polish in the many drafts that followed.

Writing a series of connected works presents certain opportunities and challenges. There's an opportunity to explore characters over several books, showing their evolution through an extended character arc. A protagonist may be a vastly different person in the final book compared to who they were in the first book. Likewise there's the chance to explore themes throughout several books, providing depth and breadth of coverage, and allowing themes to become layered and build over multiple narratives. Exploring Tess, Jack, Omar, and the other characters over several novels, as well as the different dimensions of love and the other thematic content, was a rewarding experience that allowed for character growth and thematic exploration that would not have otherwise been possible. A serial also allows for writerly tidbits that are not possible in a one-off book. For example, you can place a clue at the end of each book that signals the topic of the next book, something I did in this series.

There are also unique challenges in writing a series. You must pay attention to the narrative arc of each story and also create an overarching narrative arc across the books. Achieving this takes some planning. To accomplish the task, I used the same organization for each book, I centered each book around at least one traumatic event (although the events differed widely), and I employed a bit of "recap" in each novel, referencing important parts of earlier books. Weaving themes across titles is also important and is a part of creating an overarching narrative arc. One way I attempted to do so was by balancing drama, trauma, and humor in all the titles. This balancing of darkness and light mirrors the very journey of the characters and creates consistency across the books. When the series begins, Tess begins to learn to live with darkness and light, learning to balance the two later in the series, and eventually learning to live in color. Each novel has its own story arc, but taken together, there is a larger narrative.

A final piece of advice: always leave the door open to writing more. No matter how much you plan out a serial and design the overall narrative arc, determining how many stories that it will take to unfold, you never know when more inspiration will strike. These are characters you'll have gotten to know intimately, and so there's always the possibility you'll wish to return to their world. While I'm happy where Tess and Jack are left in *North Star*, I knew another novel was possible, and I even planted a clue at the end of the fifth book, signaling the topic for the next one.

Although I took time off and focused on other projects, partly because of the time afforded me by the 2020/2021 pandemic, I did return to these characters to write a sixth story, *Stardust*. I released new versions of all six novels in the collection *Celestial Bodies: The Tess Lee and Jack Miller Novels* (Leavy, 2022). The collection completes this work, and if you're interested in reading the series it is the version I recommend.

> Readers expect closure at the end of a novel. They like the story resolved, questions answered, and characters situated. This expectation is amplified when they've taken a journey across several books. Giving your narrative an ending doesn't have to make it final. You can create closure while still leaving open the possibility of returning to your characters. You may feel done with them now, but one thing I've learned over the years is that the creative process is not linear and inspiration doesn't always oblige our plans. Make room for all possibilities.

SKILL-BUILDING EXERCISE Based on the topic you've been working on, determine one central theme for your fictional work. Next, create a list of five possible metaphors you could use to explore that theme. Don't fret too much. In practice, most of them may not work. This is simply meant to help you begin to think metaphorically. Next, using your protagonist's journey, create a list of five possible ways to weave symbolism into the narrative and to reveal something about your character. Again, don't overthink it. This is simply meant to help you begin to think symbolically.

RETHINK YOUR RESEARCH Take one of the primary themes to emerge from your data and begin to think about it metaphorically. Create a list of five possible metaphors you could use to explore that theme. Select the strongest metaphor and write for at least 30 minutes. To do so, start writing a scene with your protagonist in which the metaphor emerges. Once you have a draft of the scene, read it and see if there is any way to weave symbolism into the scene in order to underscore the theme.

7 Alternative Structures

> Techniques highlighted in this chapter:
> ✓ Dialogue
> ✓ Internal dialogue/interiority
> ✓ Plot/story line

In the last few chapters, I've reviewed traditional three-act structures and open structures (either of which can be used for stand-alone novels, sequels, trilogies, or series). There are innumerable possibilities that exist in between these two structures. I view **alternative structures** as any model outside of conventional three-, four-, or five-part structures or wholly open structures with no prescribed format. They may be existing structures or entirely new ones that you create.

There are some alternative structures that novelists use fairly commonly. For example, a narrative can be structured as a **before-and-after story**. In this kind of narrative, there is a critical event, and the story unfolds both before *and* after the event. It is a specific way of organizing a story in two parts. An example from popular literature is *Looking for Alaska* by John Green, in which the story unfolds before and after the mysterious death of the title character.

Another commonly used alternative structure unfolds as a **before–together–after story**, in which the characters are shown individually, living their own lives, usually only briefly (in a few chapters or less). Most of the narrative then unfolds as all the characters are together (e.g., at an event such as a wedding or funeral, on vacation, in a disaster). The final and third part, again generally brief, shows the characters returning to their own lives. This way of structuring a story shows the impact that a group being together has on the characters when they return to their own lives. We have seen them before, then something happens when they are together, and then we see how they have been affected. I used this structure in my forthcoming novel *The Location Shoot* (Leavy, in press), in which a group of famous actors are each shown in their own lives, each facing a personal crossroad (e.g., a failed romance, the desire to have a child, a health challenge). Most of the novel then unfolds as they live and work together for 3 months on location in Sweden making a film that asks the big questions about the meaning of life. In the final chapter, they all return to their own lives. Inspired by their experience together, each makes a bold choice about how to deal with their personal crises.

Another alternative structure is the **multiple viewpoint narrative**. This type of story is told by changing narrator viewpoint, chapter by chapter. In the simplest version, there are two characters whose perspectives are emphasized, and these perspectives are switched from chapter to chapter. For example, popular novelist Meg Donahue has used this structure in numerous works. In her novel *How to Eat a Cupcake*, which follows two female friends, there's a chapter titled "Annie" written from Annie's perspective, followed by one titled "Julia" written from Julia's perspective, and the story continues to go back and forth in this manner. This narrative can be expanded to include more characters. For example, in Donahue's later novel *All the Summer Girls*, she uses the same structure but with three characters. A multiple viewpoint narrative can be even more complex. For example, social fiction author J. E. Sumerau's novel *Via Chicago*, which explores creating families of choice amid trauma recovery, is written from the perspectives of eight characters. The sequencing of their chapters is

> When writing a multiple viewpoint novel, it's important to clearly distinguish character voices—to make each one stand out as identifiable so that it's easy for readers to know who is narrating (e.g., consider their sense of humor, language choice, commonly used phrases, personality). Characters should be finely drawn, and each have unique voice. For added reader ease, you can label chapters with the character names. You still have to do the heavy lifting of writing well-drawn characters. Using some shorthand doesn't give you a shortcut.

unpredictable as well. So when adapting this structure, there are more and less formulaic approaches you can take, depending on your goals.

A final, widely used alternative structure is the **single-day or multiple-day narrative,** which are stories that unfold deliberately over the course of one day or a series of days (usually up to one week). With respect to the single-day narrative, there are many famous examples with which you may be familiar, including *Mrs. Dalloway* by Virginia Woolf, written largely as stream of consciousness. For a different approach to the single-day narrative, consider *The Hours* by Michael Cunningham, which is inspired by *Mrs. Dalloway.* The story follows three women at different historical times, each over the course of one day. So it is a single day for each character, but not a single day in the conventional sense. Novelists can always play with conventions. Cunningham used the single-day formula to reinforce the theme of the book, that a woman's whole life can be known by exploring a single day. Here we see a marriage between content and form. There are also many cases in which an author will tell a story over several days, which is still finite, but longer than the single-day exploration. For example, a novel I'm writing called *Shadow Harbor* unfolds over 7 days. The novel features seven parts—labeled "Tuesday," "Wednesday," and so forth, ending with "Monday." Each part, or day, unfolds over several chapters. I review this structure further in a discussion of my novel *Spark* (Leavy, 2019b).

This is by no means an exhaustive review of alternative structures. For example, the **story within a story** (also referred to as an **embedded narrative** or **nested story**) is a popular convention. There are also **fractured narratives,** which are told in a nonlinear manner (and may be particularly powerful for stories centered on trauma, depression, addiction, or other topics people are likely to experience in a nonlinear manner). And on and on. Perhaps most exciting of all, there are also the new structures you may create. Structures give shape to the stories we aim to tell. They should align with the themes and tone of the fictional work. Aim for synergy between the form and content. Ask yourself: How can I best deliver the intended content to readers? The possibilities are limited only by our imaginations.

Spark

Many years ago, I began to wonder if there was a way to combine my passion for the research process and my love of fiction. I thought about writing a novel that explores the relationship between the research process, collaboration, and critical thinking. Despite stewing on the idea on and off for years, I ultimately concluded there was no way to write a novel on the topic and make it a good piece of literary art. After all, who would want to read a novel about the research process, and how on earth would I write it? I abandoned the idea and went on to write other works of fiction, several of which have been included in this book.

Then one day out of the blue, I received an invitation. It was such an unusual invitation that my assistant, in forwarding the email, said, "This is either spam or the coolest invitation you've ever received." It wasn't spam. It was an invitation from the famed Salzburg Global Seminar in Austria, which was started in 1947 as a response to the atrocities of World War II. Since its inception, the Salzburg Global Seminar has brought scholars, activists, artists, and others from around the world to participate in sessions on various topics of import. I was one of 50 people invited to participate in Session 547 "The Neuroscience of Art: What are the Sources of Creativity and Innovation?" which was conducted February 21–26, 2015. The seminar took place at Schloss Leopoldskron, a historic castle and hotel, where the exteriors of *The Sound of Music* were shot. There were neuroscientists, artists, journalists, and scholars among us. We spent our days in breakout groups debating topics and in large lectures learning from one another. There were many heated conversations as you might expect would occur with strangers from such wide-ranging disciplines and backgrounds. Nights were spent socializing, usually into the wee hours—eating lavish spreads of food, drinking, playing ping-pong and other games in the pub, being entertained, and entertaining one another. It was an extraordinary experience. And despite our differences, we bonded as friends, and the group continues to stay in touch. Many of us have since collaborated. During my time in Salzburg, I finally figured out how to write a novel about the research process. When my husband and I traveled to Vienna after the seminar ended, I wrote the entire outline for *Spark* in my hotel room.

Spark follows Professor Peyton Wilde. Although she has an enviable life teaching sociology at an idyllic liberal arts college, she is troubled by a sense of fading inspiration. One day an invitation arrives. Peyton has been selected to attend a luxurious all-expense-paid seminar in Iceland, where participants, billed as some of the greatest thinkers in the world, will be charged with answering one perplexing question. The 49 participants are put into groups of 7. When she meets her diverse teammates—two neuroscientists, a philosopher, a dance teacher, a collage artist, and a farmer—Peyton wonders what she could ever have to contribute. The novel unfolds over the 5 days the group spends in Iceland—working on answering the dumbfounding question, socializing in the evenings, and taking day trips to famous sites where they experience the country's unique natural landscape. The ensuing journey of discovery transforms the characters' work, their biases, and ultimately themselves. In the end, they are able to answer the question that had baffled them.

The following excerpt takes place during an outing. After a morning trip to the geysers, the group has lunch together and then journeys to a waterfall. At this point, the group has accomplished little more than arguing, each one limited to their own perspective. They are still trying to unravel the meaning of the question they have been charged with answering.

Spark, Excerpt from Chapter 8

As the van approached a small hotel where they were to have lunch, everyone else was looking at trinkets they bought at the geyser gift shop—magnets, postcards, jewelry, and books, while Peyton was deep in thought. *How will we ever make progress answering the question? We saw such beauty today. And everyone's getting along. I wish I could enjoy it more. Ronnie being out of commission is making it harder. Maybe lunch will be our chance to talk, all of us as a group. I wonder if anyone will bring it up.*

"And here we are," Aldar said. The unassuming gray stucco building didn't look like much. "This hotel has a nice lunch spot with gorgeous views. Please go inside. They're expecting you. I'll be at the van when you're ready."

Everyone hopped out and made their way inside. There wasn't a soul in sight, just a small, unwatched reception desk.

"There's a sign, the restaurant is this way," Liev said, heading to the right.

They arrived in an airy, casual dining area, featuring a long wall of glass windows overlooking rolling green hills. The view was again unlike any of the others they had seen. They stood awkwardly, clearing their throats and making other innocuous noises to signal their presence. A rotund woman with honey blonde curls crashed through the swinging kitchen doors.

"Well forgive me. I hope you haven't been waiting long. You're the group from Crystal Manor, yes?"

"Yes," Liev and Dietrich replied in unison.

"Wonderful, I'm Birta. We're putting the final touches on your lunch. Please, go seat yourselves at that large table by the window. Best view in the place," she said before running off.

"How odd we're the only ones here," Peyton said.

"It's late for lunch," Liev said.

"Maybe they closed for our group," Harper mused.

By the time they seated themselves, Birta was rushing over with a pitcher of water.

"What can I get you each to drink? We have soda, juice, wine, beer, coffee, and tea."

Oh, I hope no one orders alcohol, Peyton thought. *They won't want to work.*

"I'll have a beer, please," Dietrich said.

"Me too," Liev said.

"Make it three," Milton said.

"When in Rome," Harper joined in.

Well, maybe it's a good thing. Maybe it will loosen them up, Peyton rationalized before she, Ariana, and Ronnie said they were fine with water.

They sat for a moment enjoying the serene view.

"Looks like it could be a golf course," Harper said. "Wonder if it is."

"I doubt it," Liev said.

Peyton noticed Ronnie was quiet. "You feel okay?" she whispered.

"Yeah. I'm just really disappointed I missed so much."

Birta came bursting through the kitchen doors again, with a man in cook's clothing behind her. They delivered their drinks, a loaf of bread, and a large bowl of salad.

"We prepared a family-style lunch for you. We'll bring the rest out in a minute. I know there are allergy concerns. Fear not, it's all gluten and lactose free. Even the bread."

"That's nice," Peyton said. Ronnie nodded.

Moments later Birta and the cook returned with roast chicken surrounded by potatoes and root vegetables and a platter of slow-cooked arctic char topped with microgreens.

Dietrich offered to walk around the table with the platter of chicken so everyone could help themselves.

"Lovely they made it family-style," Harper said as she passed the salad.

"Really homey," Ariana added.

The food smelled delicious. Even Ronnie took a chicken thigh and potatoes.

Everyone was enjoying their first few bites when Peyton again began to wonder if anyone would bring up the question. *Doesn't seem like they will. I should say something. But . . .*

Ariana interrupted her thoughts when she said, "This is a great opportunity to break bread together. Perhaps we should use this time to talk about the question."

Peyton looked to see their reactions before jumping in. "I agree. Let's make the most of the time we have together."

"Good idea," Harper said.

"Yes, let's be productive," Liev concurred.

"How should we begin?" Ariana asked.

They sat, the only noise the sound of chewing. A couple of minutes passed before Ronnie said, "Maybe we should tackle it indirectly. Then tomorrow back at the lodge we can take a more direct approach."

Peyton smiled, unable to hide her joy that Ronnie was participating again.

"I had a thought," Harper said.

"Yes, what is it?" Dietrich asked.

"Might be nothing but I'm wondering if it's important they put us in groups of seven. It's not fifty participants, it's forty-nine."

"I noticed the number seven was a part of a larger number on my welcome packet. I think it was seven at least," Peyton said.

Ariana nodded. "The number seven has a rich history. Perhaps if we talk about it we'll stumble on to something."

Everyone seemed to agree.

"Should someone take notes?" Ariana asked before eating a bite of carrots.

"I think we can be informal and let everyone enjoy lunch," Liev said.

Peyton took a small notebook and pen out of her bag. "I don't mind jotting a few things down."

"Maybe we should start by listing the most obvious things that come to mind. Then we can see how it develops," Ariana suggested.

"Sounds good," Ronnie said. "I'm happy to get us going. What first comes to mind for me is the seven continents."

Ariana smiled. "For Americans that's a good example, but there's a cultural element to geography and what is considered a continent. It's not universal."

Hmm. Peyton thought. *That's interesting. We are an international group. Maybe we should talk about that.* But the moment escaped her.

"There are seven seas," Milton said.

"And seven wonders of the world," Harper said. "Oh, and something in music too, uh ... "

Dietrich smiled. "There are seven distinct notes in the diatonic musical scale," he said.

"Yes!" Harper exclaimed.

"There are seven holes in the human head," Milton said before asking Liev to pass the potatoes.

"That's funny. I never thought of that," Harper said.

"I'm sure there's a good joke in there," Ariana mused.

"Seven is considered a lucky number," Peyton said.

"Yeah, when you roll two dice, seven has the highest probability of coming up," Ronnie said.

"Slot machines pay off with triple sevens," Milton added.

Harper looked at him curiously.

"My wife and I go to Atlantic City sometimes," he said.

Harper smiled. "Do you get saltwater taffy? I loved that stuff as a kid."

"I like the peppermint," Peyton said.

Milton shook his head. "Too chewy. Never touch it."

Ronnie chimed in, "You know, to go in a bit of a different direction if that's okay, one of the first things that I thought of hearing the number seven was popular culture. Maybe it's different in other places, but in American pop culture seven appears a lot in films, books, and so on."

"I think it holds true to some extent," Ariana said. "*Harry Potter* comes to mind. Seven is important in those books. And with the prominence of Hollywood we're probably all exposed to many of the same things, for better or worse."

Dietrich agreed. "I admit I enjoy the James Bond movies, 007."

Harper smiled.

They all continued eating and everyone began listing books and movies from William Shakespeare to Neil Gaiman. After twenty minutes, they had full bellies but were running short on ideas. Birta came to clear the dishes and serve coffee, tea, and a small tray of pastel-colored macaroons.

"May I say something?" Dietrich asked.

"Go ahead," Milton said.

"When I hear the number seven what comes to my mind is religion. Seven is an important number in many religions. Of course the Old Testament says that the world was created in seven days, the seventh being the day of rest."

"Yes," Peyton said. "In Kabbalah it says that because God rested on the seventh day he added a spiritual dimension to the world. Seven is considered a spiritual number."

Liev concurred. "For the record, I don't think any of this seven discussion is relevant but nevertheless Christianity is full of references to seven: deadly sins, gifts from God, sacraments."

Dietrich nodded. "In Revelation, the Seventh Angel will blow the seventh trumpet seven times and a lamb will break open the seven seals to reveal the mystery of God."

"Seven is prominent in other religions too. I can think of examples in Hinduism, Taoism, and Judaism," Ariana said.

Harper said, "It's not just organized religions. I'm not religious. I've read a lot about New Age spirituality though."

Liev pursed his lips.

Harper continued. "Seven is the path of introspection according to some."

"I think we've taken this as far as we can, talking in circles," Liev said.

"I want to mention one other thing," Harper said. "Seven shows up in mythology too."

Liev rubbed his eyes, visibly losing his patience.

"Tell us more," Ronnie said.

"Atlas had seven daughters. They helped populate the heavens. Zeus turned them into a seven star configuration," Harper said.

"We've reached fantasy at this point. Mythology is nonsense," Liev shrieked.

"Not everyone feels that way. Perhaps you're just a bit closed minded," Harper rebuffed.

"I did not want to say this earlier but if seven is important, it's because of neuroscience," Liev said.

"Well gee, that's a novel conclusion for you!" Ronnie exclaimed.

"It is the truth. There is a neurological basis for humans' preference for seven. We can generally remember seven-digit numbers, not eight. It's quite simple. Our brains are best able to store the number seven. If the number seven is some sort of clue, it is pointing us back to science, as I have said from day one."

Everyone was speechless. Milton picked up his coffee cup and slurped his last sip, breaking the silence.

Birta came over and asked, "Can I get you anything else?"

Peyton shook her head. "I think we're done."

* * *

"Gullfoss is Europe's most powerful waterfall. It's one of the natural wonders of the world," Aldar said as he parked the van.

"Is it a protected site?" Ariana asked.

"Yes. It is a designated nature reserve," Aldar replied. "When you walk over you will see it is split into upper and lower waterfalls. There's a staircase, and I recommend you venture up to the top to experience every view. You will also notice the color of the water is remarkable and changes in different lighting. The magic of glacial water. Please return to the van when you're done. There's no rush."

Everyone got out and started walking toward the massive crashing waterfall. It wasn't until they were close that they realized a large crevice had been obscured from view and the water was plummeting into a canyon below.

"Wow! It's spectacular," Harper said.

"Awe-inspiring," Ariana said.

Everyone took photographs for a few minutes before Liev said, "Shall we follow the lower path and then head up to the top?"

Peyton looked at the steep staircase off to the left and began to panic. *I can't believe how high it is. I can't go up there,* she thought, but she said nothing. They began following the lower path, toward the thunderous sound of crashing water.

"The mist feels good," Harper said.

Peyton smiled. "The color is beautiful. I've never seen water like this."

"It's because of the sediments in glacial water," Milton said.

"How do you know so much about it?" Harper asked.

"Nature enthusiast. That's my life."

"That's interesting about the sediments," Ronnie said. "Can you tell us more?"

Milton regaled the group with his vast knowledge of different kinds of water all the way to the end of the path.

They were taking pictures when Ariana said, "Seeing how unique the glacial water is makes me think about the glaciers."

"Peyton really wants to visit some of the glaciers," Ronnie said.

Peyton smiled. "Yeah, maybe someday."

Liev put his phone in his pocket and turned to Peyton. "Someday is always in the distance. Someday is dangerous. Be careful of someday."

Peyton felt like he could see right through her. *I can't believe he said that to me, like he knows I'll never get there. He's probably right too.* Unsure of how to respond, she was relieved when Dietrich said, "The glaciers may not exist someday if humans do not make serious changes. I know Icelanders are rightfully concerned."

Ariana nodded. "Exactly what I was thinking," she said. "It's especially sad for people living in more ecologically responsible cultures to be at the mercy of those countries who do not care. We all share this one planet. The many have their fate sealed by the few."

Harper chimed in, "What I don't understand is the CEOs of these companies and the politicians who support them have families too. Don't they worry for their grandchildren's futures?"

"They don't believe in science," Liev said. "They are stuck in their dinosaur mentality."

Ronnie nodded. "It is dinosaur thinking. That dinosaur thinking will be their end. It's gonna eat 'em for lunch one day."

"And all of us too, I fear, if we don't find a new way to think," Ariana said.

Dinosaur thinking. A new way to think. Hmm. Peyton thought before drifting back to Liev's earlier comment. *I wonder why he said that to me about someday. It's like he sees my hesitance. Is he judging me?* Liev's voice broke her stream of consciousness.

"Okay, shall we head back and go to the upper level?" he asked.

Oh no, I really can't go up there. I mean, I kind of want to, but I can't.

* * *

A few minutes later they were standing at the base of a precipitous staircase. Peyton looked up with dread. Her heart began to beat faster. *Maybe it's not as high as it seems*, she rationalized. Just as Liev was about to step up, Peyton panicked and blurted out, "I'm gonna wait down here. I don't want to go up there."

Liev turned around and asked, "Why not? What's the problem?"

Harper replied, "She's afraid of heights. Remember?"

"Ah, it's perfectly safe," Liev insisted.

"Our fears aren't always rational," Dietrich said.

I'm so embarrassed. I can't believe this is becoming such a big deal, Peyton thought.

"If you don't feel comfortable, there's no pressure," Ariana said. Peyton tilted her head. "Thank you. I just ... I just ... "

"Hey," Ronnie said, rubbing Peyton's arm. "I'm still pretty low energy. I can stay down here with you."

"Oh, no. You missed so much already. Please go," Peyton said. "I actually sort of want to go too, it's just that I'm worried I'll start up and be too scared. I don't want to get stuck."

The corners of Liev's mouth turned upward ever so slightly, offering her the subtlest of smiles. "If you would like to overcome your fear, now is a good time. I will walk behind you. If you are too afraid, stop and turn around. I'll lead you back down," he said.

Peyton imagined how beautiful the view would be and that it was likely her only chance to see it, so she agreed.

The group slowly made their way up the staircase, along with other tourists. Liev kept his promise, following Peyton and reminding her they could head back if needed. In the beginning she was anxious, her palms sweaty and mind racing, but she took deep breaths at the suggestion of Harper and Ariana. Contrary to her fear, the higher they got, the less nervous she felt. By the time they reached the top, she was exhilarated. As she took the last step up, the group began clapping. Peyton blushed. She turned to Liev and said, "Thank you." He smiled and said, "You're quite welcome. Today is always better than someday."

They all walked to the spot with the clearest view.

"We should take a group picture," Harper suggested. She handed her phone to Dietrich. "Your arms are longer than mine."

They smooshed together for a group selfie.

"I'll send it to all of you," Harper said.

"It's really spectacular, isn't it?" Ronnie said.

Everyone agreed.

"And look," Harper said. "There are so many rainbows."

Peyton grinned like a Cheshire cat. "Rainbows have seven colors."

Reflection on *Spark*

Spark is a short and simple novel, but it was challenging to write. There weren't readily available models. Its unique premise and goals gave me little to draw from when trying to figure out how to write it. It's also largely based on seven people in conversation together. Writing dialogue for a group that size is challenging since fiction typically centers on conversations between fewer characters. Focusing on seven characters required them to be clearly distinguished from each other from the outset. Characters were finely drawn, with each one's perspective and personality becoming clear from the start. I used a mix of dialogue, interiority, and narrator commentary in order to show who each person is, how they see themselves, and how the others see them.

Deciding to employ a framework whereby the narrative unfolds over a predetermined number of days enabled me to structure the story. I determined what insights would need to occur each day in order for the group to arrive at the eventual answer, concluding their journey and the book. In the preceding extract, while every word carries meaning, there were four developments that needed to occur. First, Ariana, the only person of color in the group, was largely ignored at lunch when she mentioned the cultural aspect to things we take for granted. This happens repeatedly throughout the novel, although as we learn in the end, her insights were critical. Second, the concept of outdated or "dinosaur" thinking needed to surface. This is a breadcrumb left for readers that becomes increasingly important to solving the problem. Next, I wanted to raise the idea that "today is better than someday," a recurrent theme in the book. Finally, at the end of the chapter, Peyton remarks that rainbows have seven colors, just like their group. This is a metaphor or even a simple reminder that together human beings create something larger than the sum of their individual selves. The structure I imposed, with the narrative occurring over 5 days, not only helped me clarify *when* each insight would naturally surface, but also *how* each one would occur. In other words, the structure helped me develop the plot and story line. For example, when you only have 5 days to work with, meals become an important time. Given that the book centers on a group of seven strangers trying to work together across glaring differences, the concept of "breaking bread" as a time for coming together made sense and I used it to the fullest. It's during the more informal conversations during meals that some of the most important developments take place.

Now when I think back to my initial idea many years ago of writing a novel about knowledge building and problem solving, I realize that without figuring out that it needed to unfold over just a few days, I could never have done it. Stumbling on the right structure was the only way to figure out the ensuing story and to tell it in a way that might be engaging for readers. I had never written a novel like *Spark* before, and in some ways, I doubt I will again. Subject-wise, it's a one-off. It was an experiment, and I'm pleased with the result. Pushing myself to write in a different way was invaluable for me as a writer. I'm much more likely and better equipped to play with different ways of structuring a story, and in that way, for me, *Spark* was not an ending, but a beginning. I encourage you to try different ways of telling your stories. The more you do so, the more you'll realize there are that many more stories you can tell.

SKILL-BUILDING EXERCISE Take the plot and story line you wrote at the end of Chapter 4 and write a new plot and story line using an alternative structure. Once you have completed the new plot and structure, compare it to the traditional three-act plot and story line you created. Write a one- to two-page response to how structuring the narrative differently changes how you tell the story. Which structure better suits your project?

RETHINK YOUR RESEARCH Take the plot and story line you wrote at the end of Chapter 4 and write a new plot and story line using an alternative structure. Consider the way you garnered data and the nature of that data as you determine which structure to use. For example, if you conducted interviews or oral history interviews with participants, consider a multiple-viewpoint narrative. If you conducted ethnographic field research, consider a single-day or multiple-day narrative, meant to mirror an in-depth look into your field site and participants' lives. If you are working on a sensitive topic, such as trauma, domestic abuse, or homelessness, consider a fractured narrative. These are just examples.

8 Short Stories

> Techniques highlighted in this chapter:
> ✓ Names
> ✓ Dialogue
> ✓ Internal dialogue/interiority
> ✓ Symbolism

So far, I've reviewed different ways of structuring a novel, a full-length literary work. Novels typically range from 40,000 to over 100,000 words.[1] However, sometimes we want to write shorter works of fiction. **Novellas** are literary works that typically range from 10,000 to 40,000 words. **Short stories** are generally 1,000 to 10,000 words long.[2] They are works of fiction that rely on the same literary techniques used for novels, but they can be read in one sitting and have a more succinct narrative. Short stories may be published individually in literary magazines or journals or may be presented in collections, either in a collection by a single author or in an anthology featuring the work of numerous authors. Some writers begin their journey into creative writing with short stories. It makes sense because they require mastery of the same literary tools as a novel, but they may feel more manageable. I do want to caution though that writing something shorter is not necessarily easier. Whether you choose this structure depends on the kind of writer you are.

Low-Fat Love Stories

After my novel *Low-Fat Love* was released, I was bombarded with messages from readers telling me how the novel affected them. I was routinely stopped in hallways after book talks or conference presentations. Strangers would whisper their incredibly personal stories of low-fat love to me. Some shared stories of divorce, domestic violence, sexual assault, eating disorders, alcoholism, dysfunctional relationships, heartbreak, grief, depression, and attempted suicide. The protagonist in the novel, Prilly, hit a nerve with readers. I think the book tapped into the loneliness many feel as they struggle with different versions of low-fat love.

As readers shared their stories with me, I learned more about the concept of low-fat love or of settling in life and in love. I wanted to honor this new learning. These informal conversations and reader notes prompted me to conduct a new set of qualitative interviews. I explicitly sought out women across the age spectrum and from different backgrounds with respect to race, ethnicity, religion, sexuality, education, and profession. These interviews, conducted via email so that I could reach a broad range of women, centered on dissatisfying relationships, past or present, with a romantic partner, family member, or even with themselves. "Dissatisfying" was not defined for the women, allowing each of them to interpret the term in her own way. The stories focus on settling in relationships, toxic dynamics, the gap between fantasies and realities, recognizing and breaking relationship patterns, feeling like a fraud, going through divorce, experiencing abuse, spirituality, recovering from childhood trauma, having poor body image, aging, and more. It is those interviews that became the basis for a collection of 16 short stories, *Low-Fat Love Stories*.

> I'm not a believer in the concept of "writer's block." Sometimes writing is hard, and we have to work for each word. That's when discipline matters. Discipline is the antidote to so-called writer's block. However, sometimes we lack inspiration, and cross-pollination or collaboration can fuel us. If you're having trouble determining a direction for your work, seek out other writers, scholars, or artists and run your ideas by them. Sometimes they'll come up with something you never would have thought of on your own.

The stories interviewees shared were raw, layered, and deeply emotional. I had visceral reactions reading them and was moved to tears many times. My goal was to honor the texture and tone of what each woman shared. I originally intended to write this book alone. I had already collected and analyzed the data but felt "stuck" and unsure of how to proceed. Looking for some inspiration, I invited creative arts therapist and visual artist Victoria Scotti to collaborate. Victoria was the ideal collaborator; she also qualitatively studied women's lives, but as a visual artist she had a different approach and perspective. She thought about things differently. Together we worked with the purpose of authentically transmitting the women's stories in a way that would allow readers their own visceral, emotional, and intellectual responses.

How were the stories constructed? After immersing myself in the interview transcripts and engaging in qualitative analysis, I created a summary of each interview that included demographic information about the participant, themes that emerged, and a selection of key quotations. I sent each summary to Victoria. Based on the summary she created a "visual concept" meant to represent the essence of the interview—the theme, texture, and tone. I then used the visual art as inspiration for writing each story. Drawing directly on verbatim interview transcripts as well as on my imagination, I drafted each story. Generally about half of the words in the stories are direct language from the interview. I kept the first-person narration to bring readers into the minds and experiences of the women. Each woman was assigned a pseudonym. When writing these stories, I employed a range of different styles—diary entries, interior monologue, or constructed scenes or conversations—so there is variation within the collection.

As noted earlier in this book, there is a wide-reaching continuum regarding how social fiction is created, from practices whereby the act of writing is the method of inquiry and methods that are drawn more directly from traditional qualitative research practice. As a novelist, I tend to use writing as my method of inquiry. I have included an example from *Low-Fat Love Stories* because it developed from a qualitative practice and it differs from the other exemplars in this book. It thus serves as an example of transforming qualitative data garnered from a conventional method into a fictional work. Qualitative data were collected and then analyzed using traditional strategies. The visual art served as an additional layer of analysis. After both rounds of analysis, the stories were developed, drawn directly from participants' own language. The process of writing was an act of interpretation and representation. Again this process is very similar to a traditional qualitative methodology and could just as easily be employed to develop a longer work, such as a novella or novel. Moreover, although in this project we added a layer of visual analysis, one could move directly from traditional coding to fictional writing (see Figure 8.1).

In the following story, I combined the interviews of two women in order to create a fictional meeting and conversation that focuses on how these women feel about themselves and how they perceive they appear to others. Eleanor is 59 years old, white, and identifies as a lesbian. Mary is also 59 years old, white, and did not disclose her sexual orientation. Although given the opportunity, neither woman disclosed her religious preference.

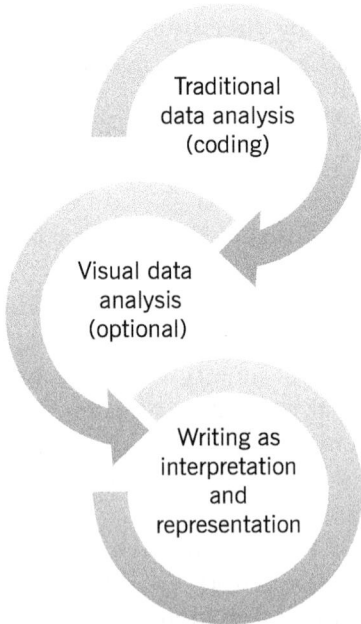

FIGURE 8.1 The process of moving from qualitative data to fictional writing.

Low-Fat Love Stories, Chapter 10, "Mirror Mirror"

Eleanor

If the hotel lobby is any indication, the conference will be packed. I hope it trickles into my book signing. Sometimes I think women are afraid to be seen buying a book about female orgasm. Pretty sad. We can't even be interested in our own bodies without shame. Hmm... which way is my room? This place is like a maze. God, I hope Mary turns out to be a decent roommate. Rooming with a stranger is always scary. Just let me feel safe. Please don't let her be a homophobe. It's exhausting being guarded all the time. She seemed fine on email, but I'll bet she says something about my appearance. Why do they always think they can do that? It's so invasive. I'm butch, get over it. Hold up, Eleanor. Don't get ahead of yourself. Just because the last one was bad doesn't mean Mary will be. Don't prejudge her. Maybe she'll be swell. Give her a chance. Ah, here's the room.

* * *

Mary

Maybe I shouldn't have unpacked before Eleanor is here. I hope she's not offended I took the bed by the window. I don't know if she gets up in the middle of the night so I was trying to be considerate giving her the bed by the bathroom. What if she thinks it's rude? I don't know why I get nervous in these situations. For Christ's sake, Mary, you preach empowerment to women. And she seemed nice over email. I'm giving so many lectures at the conference I'll hardly be in the room anyway. It'll be fine. I'm curious too. Her work is so bold. I wonder what she looks like. She's probably a powerhouse. She'll probably look at me like a little old lady compared to her. Oh my goodness, I think she's here.

* * *

Eleanor and Mary

"Hi, you must be Eleanor. I'm Mary. Welcome."

"Nice to meet you, Mary."

"I hope you don't mind I took this bed. I left the drawers over there empty."

"Okay, thanks. I'm going to try to unpack quickly, before I go down to the book exhibit."

"I have to confess that when I put my name in the conference roommate-finder portal, I was a little worried about who I would get matched with. I've experienced a range in the past, but I do like to share hotel costs when I speak at these conventions. As soon as they sent me your information I looked you up and was blown away by your latest book. Holy moly!"

"Common reaction, Mary. Most people don't expect someone our age, let alone someone who looks like me, to write about female orgasm."

"True, people don't think women our age care about orgasms. I'm curious, do readers expect you to be younger? When you give talks at conventions like this are people generally surprised by what you look like?"

"Probably some are. I'm fairly certain that most people who see me on the street assume that I am an asexual kind of person, both because I look butch and because I look older. I doubt anyone pegs me for a sex and intimacy expert."

"How do people react when they find out about your work?"

"Most are surprised. Some are curious, others seem frightened off."

"Is it hard to, you know, meet people?"

"The fact that I have so many opinions about sex intimidates people who might otherwise be interested in dating, I think."

"I can see that, Eleanor."

"To be honest, though, the age thing puts women off too. Maybe more than anything else. Fifty-nine is tough."

"It sure is. I don't usually talk about this with people, I can't in my circles, but as I'm nearing 60 I feel pretty terrible about the way I look."

"What bothers you, Mary?"

"I'm 20 pounds heavier than I'd like to be. Some women look like a young 60, but I feel like the extra pounds make me more matronly."

"My body isn't as trim as it once was either, Mary, and sometimes I miss that."

"I felt bad about my weight most of my life. I remember starting to feel this way when I was around eight. People can say such cruel things. I remember being told 'nobody loves a fatty,' and 'you'd be so pretty if you lost weight.' I've been on a diet or off a diet ever since."

"That's awful. I'm sorry."

"Eleanor, can I tell you something I've never told a soul? A few years ago I went through the horrible realization that even if I were able to lose the weight I'd struggled with since I was a girl, I'd still have wrinkles and look old."

"I'll bet most women our age can relate. An enormous number of women feel inadequate and make themselves miserable. When you look like me, you learn the importance of self-acceptance early on. I mean, I'm a butch dyke—butcher than any of those portrayed on TV, as you can see. So it's not like I buy into the toxic pop culture where women are portrayed as automatons. But the age thing even gets me. Sometimes when I see myself in the mirror, or when I see myself through others' eyes, I feel bad about the way I look."

"Oh, Eleanor, I don't like looking in mirrors either. Seeing someone unattractive looking back is terrible. Part of what makes me suffer is the mismatch of how I feel I look and the mirror's confrontation."

"Exactly."

"How I imagine I look to others is even worse. My husband doesn't know this because he would focus on why I care how other men see me, but about four years ago I had the 'invisible experience.' That was incredibly painful. As I've aged, the number of men who notice me has dwindled, but now it's as if they would rather not see me at all. It doesn't matter that I have a spouse. There's a profound feeling of loss, of erasure, when it becomes clear men are not open to the flirting I have done most of my life."

"For me, I feel like I am seen, but it isn't necessarily me they are really seeing. It's a stereotype, it's the one-dimensional version they want me to be. Men react to any butch dyke with fear. I'm not seen as a 'real' woman, whatever that means. And women can be just as judgmental."

"How do you find women judgmental?"

"Well, my usual style for dressing is very tough, casual, and what most people consider masculine. You can't entirely tell in this environment, because when I'm working I always make an attempt to look soft and try to tone it down so I don't alienate people. But even though my style is very butch, it's fun to dress up sometimes, and occasionally I would like to dress more femininely. The main reason I don't is because I'm afraid of the comments I would get from friends who see me as a butch lesbian, and want to keep seeing me as a butch lesbian."

"It seems no matter what we look like, and what our style is, we have to contend with the expectations of others. Don't you think, Eleanor?"

"We internalize those expectations too. For the most part I really do like to wear casual things like old jeans, which fit my daily lifestyle, but I do wonder sometimes if I really dress the way I do because it makes me feel stronger and less likely to be harassed or attacked in some way. These fears and stereotypes go very deep."

"I hope you take this the right way, but it's comforting to know that I'm not alone."

"You said before that you never really share this with anyone, Mary. I guess I don't, either. I'm used to talking to women about their bodies and sexual identities, but I keep my own mostly to myself."

"I'm sure you'll relate; in my line of work, where I have a platform to coach others, I don't feel able to share these dark realities. I don't want to disappoint them, or diminish my message, even if I can't live up to it. I feel like the world sees me as a confident person and it's mostly inside that I suffer."

"If we could only block out how we think others see us, I wonder if we would see ourselves differently."

"Oh, Eleanor, I just noticed the time. We should probably get down to the conference."

"To give women empowerment lectures kind of makes you smile, doesn't it? All those eyes on us. You know, they will see us as strong and confident, Mary."

"If only I saw myself through their eyes."

"Isn't that the problem?"

* * *

Mary

Eleanor is remarkable. When I saw her, I never would have guessed we'd have anything in common. She's right that there's no one like her on TV. She's so masculine. I feel badly for how I judged her when she walked into the room. I was intimidated. I guess in some ways I'm one of those judgmental women she was taking about. That's hard to admit. I hope it wasn't obvious. Okay, focus Mary. Women who admire you are waiting. You need to be what they want to see. Get your head in the game.

* * *

Eleanor

Mary looks great for her age. Too bad she has such a hard time accepting herself. Who says to a girl, "Nobody loves a fatty" and "You'd be pretty if you lost weight." What's wrong with people? How is any girl supposed to feel good about herself? But God, if she only knew the things they said to me. Her skin would crawl. Try having "Ugly dyke, I hope you die" screamed at you on the playground or muttered under the breath of men on the subway. There are so many times I've prayed to have the invisible experience. For her it's erasure; for me it would be survival.

Reflection on *Low-Fat Love Stories*

I used a few strategies when writing this story: identifying the narrators by name and using interiority and dialogue. Because it is a short story, there's little time to develop the characters and distinguish their voices. As a method of shorthand, for reader ease, I distinguished which character's perspective we are hearing by using their names to structure the narrative. I also used interiority to show what each woman was thinking as she prepared to meet her assigned roommate. Interiority was used to quickly distinguish each character. Readers are privy to each woman's stream of consciousness—her fears, concerns, and biases. We get a sense of the gap between how others see her and how she sees herself. Most of the story then unfolds through dialogue between the women. We learn about who they are, what work is like, and the challenges they face. I concluded by returning to interiority to show the effect each woman has had on the other.

Although it's a short piece, to build thematic content I also drew on symbolism, for example, mirrors. They are used to symbolize how we see ourselves, how others see us, and our perception of how others see us. The "mismatch" Mary notes between how she thinks of herself versus what she sees in the mirror speaks directly to the concept of low-fat love guiding the book. There's a gap between what we want and what we feel we're able to get. Many of our self-esteem challenges arise from that gap. Similarly, in this story, there is a gap between how each woman feels about herself and what she believes others see.

SKILL-BUILDING EXERCISE You have everything you need to draft a complete short story. Select one of the two plotlines you created, and using the traditional three-act or alternative structure, write your story. Don't worry, this story isn't meant to be published, it's meant to help you practice the craft of writing. As with any other craft, the only way to learn is by doing it. Just write. If you find that your plot and story line can't be adequately covered in a short story–length piece, you may need to sacrifice parts of the story or challenge yourself to draft a novella or novel. Again using what you've created for the exercises throughout this book, you have all the building blocks to write a work of fiction. Go for it.

RETHINK YOUR RESEARCH You have everything you need to draft a complete short story based on your research. Select one of the two plotlines you created, and write your story, using the traditional three-act or alternative structure. Depending on whether you've already collected data and the nature of that data, you will need to decide the degree to which you will ground the fictional work in your data and the degree to which you'll incorporate your imagination. The goal isn't to publish the resulting fictional work, only to reimagine how you could use social fiction in your research and to show that you have the building blocks to do it.

NOTES

1. Whereas novels are anything over 40,000 words, note that some publishers and literary contests have their own word-count specifications—some requiring 50,000 or 60,000 minimum-word counts for adult fiction.
2. There are some short stories that are less than 1,000 words (e.g., flash fiction). There are also examples of what authors deem short stories that are as long as 15,000 words. Authors can often choose how to label these midlength pieces, as there's a blurry line between a short story and a novella.

Practical Advice for Publishing and Evaluating Social Fiction

Although I live my professional life in the halls of the academy, seeking to both learn and communicate truth, or at least truths, it is in the world of the imaginary I have most closely experienced the real.
—ULRICH TEUCHER

You've written a work of social fiction. Now what? How can you publish it? How can you support the published work? How will it be evaluated by others? Before getting into specific suggestions for getting your work out into the world, I want to return to the advice that concluded Chapter 3: develop your own relationship with your writing that isn't dependent on anything external. The literary world is highly competitive. Academia is deeply hierarchical. By doing this work, you're placing footholds in two worlds in which competition, rejection, and criticism are the norms. No matter how hard you've worked and how brilliant your writing is, it won't be liked by everyone. There will be rejections. There will be critique. So before I share strategies for publishing your work, I want to remind you that you can't control how audiences respond to it. While you're working on your story, seek feedback in the ways I suggested or in whatever ways suit you. Be ruthless with the editing process. However, once you've decided the piece is done, let it go. Make peace with it and let it go. When you're ready to do that, you're ready to publish.

Publishing Fiction

Social fiction in the form of short stories and the like are generally published in literary magazines, literary journals, or academic journals. Do an online search to find appropriate venues and follow their submission instructions carefully. Short stories can also be published as a part of an anthology (a book with contributions from multiple authors) or a collection (a book published by one author). There are also many contests for flash fiction, short stories, and other works with smaller word counts. Sometimes the prize includes publication (read contracts and/or agreements carefully so that you understand the issues related to copyright, and so forth, elaborated later). There are also online platforms, such as Submittable, that curate submission opportunities. Bear in mind that some venues require a submission fee (which does not guarantee publication).

There are four primary pathways for publishing full-length works of fiction: trade publishers, academic publishers, self-publishing, and hybrid publishers. Each has its own advantages and disadvantages.

In the world of general or commercial fiction, the most common way to publish is with a trade publisher. Trade publishers are set up to reach general readers. However, most trade publishers do not accept unsolicited submissions. Authors need a literary agent. The world of trade publishing is extremely competitive and getting an agent is no easy task. I say this in no way to discourage you, but rather to prepare you for the realities you will face. At the time of this writing, Google puts the odds of getting a literary agent as 1 out of every 6,000. Like I said, it's competitive. That does not mean you shouldn't try if you feel trade publishing is the path for you. Be prepared: some of the most famous novelists in the world say it took them many years and hundreds of rejections to get an agent. Perseverance matters. Preparedness does too. First, your book manuscript needs to be complete and professionally copyedited before you approach agents. Make it sparkle. Second, do your research. Buy the most current guide to literary agents and comb through it. Any agent who

> You can also attend writing conferences where you can meet and even pitch agents. Many literary agents get new clients this way. There are also opportunities on social media, through contests and the like, to reach out to agents. For example, check out Pitch Wars on Twitter, which hosts four pitch days per year.

accepts in your genre and is currently accepting submissions should be on your list. Going to their websites to do "extra" homework on them and the books they've published may also be helpful.

Third, write a synopsis of your book and an awesome query letter (both of which you should also have professionally copyedited). The one-page query letter should introduce your book, with a hook, and introduce you (don't be afraid to brag about your accomplishments and let your personality shine). Fourth, follow instructions. Let me repeat that, follow instructions. Some agents will want just the query letter and the first three pages of your manuscript. Some will want the letter, a synopsis, and the first 20 pages. And on and on. Send them exactly what they have requested and use the method they have specified (e.g., in the body of an email, as an email attachment, as an online submission, or as snail mail). Finally, when the inevitable silence or rejections come, find more agents, and send the material out again.

If you're successful in finding a literary agent to represent you, read your contract carefully and make sure you understand the terms. It's always advisable to have an attorney review the contract as well, if you're able to do so. Your agent will pitch your novel directly to publishers, and if the agent receives any offers, you'll be able to decide whether or not to accept them. Many fiction writers consider trade publishing the holy grail, but on the downside it's highly competitive, and authors lose a lot of control over the process.

Although generally academic publishers do not publish fiction, thanks to the recent growth in social fiction, some academic publishers have changed their policies. And you can always pitch your book even to those who don't. Someone always has to be the first. I've published social fiction with three publishers, none of whom published fiction prior to my work. If you go that route, you'll need to come up with an angle to try to sell them on the idea. You do not need an agent to pitch an academic publisher, and typically the work does not need to be complete. Publishers have different requirements that are posted on their websites, but generally you need a book proposal and a sample chapter. If you work in academia and you need your book to "count as research," then academic publishing may be ideal. It's also less competitive. You only need one publisher to say yes.

> Trade and academic publishers are commonly referred to as "traditional publishers." However, in the literary world, the term traditional publisher is generally understood to be a trade publisher.

On the downside, most academic publishers are not equipped to market to general readers, so you may end up with a far more limited potential audience. Academic publishers also generally price their books higher than trade publishers, so before you sign a deal, I suggest discussing a suitable price point. No one is going to buy an $80 novel.

Self-publishing involves authors publishing their own work. While self-publishing used to have a bad rap, there are highly professional ways to do it, and for many authors, it makes sense. When you self-publish, you retain the copyright and all the other rights to your work. There are numerous platforms that you can use to self-publish your work. One of the best known is Kindle Direct Publishing (KDP). KDP will publish your book as a paperback, hardcover, and/or e-book. The platform has online templates, and the process is relatively simple. It is also highly responsive to email inquiries from authors. With KDP, there are no up-front costs, and the royalty split favors authors. This process is enabled by print-on-demand technology, in which each paperback or hardcover is printed when ordered, so there is no costly set print run or warehousing. These days many publishers use print-on-demand technology, including some well-known academic publishers. There are other platforms that assist with self-publishing, but many charge fees and demand a print run, so explore your options carefully to see what makes the most sense given your goals. The downside of self-publishing is that you're on your own. If you go this route, I highly suggest you hire professional freelancers—at minimum a copy editor (every author needs a copy editor, not a friend, but a professional). Depending on your comfort level and budget, you may also want to hire a typesetter and cover designer. Ask colleagues for suggestions, do an online search (and then research each one), or use the list of suggestions provided by KDP. Also note that if you purchase your own ISBN at a modest cost, you can start your own imprint, and the publisher's name that appears on online retailers will be the name you have selected (as opposed to KDP or whatever platform you've used).

Hybrid publishers combine the features of trade publishing and self-publishing. There is a vetted submission process. Authors who receive acceptances usually pay a fee to cover the publishing costs (these fees can vary but are generally at least $7,500). Hybrid publishers provide many of the services that trade publishers provide, including cover design, typesetting, sales, and marketing. Authors retain the copyright and often other rights (which vary based on the publisher and what each author negotiates for their contract), and authors receive high royalties (often 60–70%, which is worlds above the 2–15% traditional publishers pay).

For those who can afford it, this is a great option for authors who want to retain legal ownership of their work and be more involved in the production and marketing process. On the downside, you must financially invest with no way of knowing if you'll see that money again. Also, although hybrid publishing has grown dramatically over the past 15 years, in part due to print-on-demand technology, and has produced many successful books, there are still those in the literary world who turn their nose up at the practice.

> A hybrid publisher is *not* the same as a vanity press. Hybrid publishers have editorial teams, and submissions are fully vetted. It's a competitive process. The best hybrid publishers accept less than 10% of submissions, sometimes much less (although they may accept more in agreements in which they develop the project and provide additional editorial services). Vanity presses are rubber stamps—they'll sign and publish just about anything. Bear in mind that whether you're seeking a literary agent and trade publisher, an academic publisher, or a hybrid publisher, if they are legitimate, there will be a rigorous submission process. The good news is that when your work is accepted, you can feel truly proud of the accomplishment. Worried about vanity or other scam presses? Do your research on any publisher before signing a deal to make sure it is reputable. Look up their recent books on the most popular online retailers. Be wary of any publisher who seeks you out. Publishing is competitive; authors go to publishers, not the other way around.

Bear in mind that if you are offered a book contract from any type of publisher, make certain you read and understand it in full, and seek professional advice as needed. If you email your editor questions about the contract, make sure you understand the full implications of the responses, and if you don't, follow up. Keep a record of these communications. Also, all terms are negotiable. While I'm not providing in-depth counsel on book contracts, I do want to mention a few clauses that may be particularly important to fiction authors.

First, the copyright. Some publishers may request transferal of the copyright, which gives them full, legal ownership of your work. Many fiction authors wish to retain copyright. Personally, I own the copyright to all but one of my works of fiction, and in that one case, I was comfortable assigning copyright to that particular publisher. As a general matter,

I would advise any author to think long and hard before signing over the copyright to their fiction. Second, derivative rights, which can include the rights to your characters. In other words, if you grant your publisher these rights, you can be prevented from writing about these characters again, including writing a sequel, a series, and so on. These rights may also extend to licensing, entertainment, and merchandising, which many fiction authors wish to retain. Third, a non-compete clause. Most book contracts have some language that speaks to the issue of non-compete clauses, in which you are prohibited from publishing another work that could compete with the sales of the existing work. These clauses need to be finely drawn, or they can prevent you from developing a body of work. For example, many novelists write in a particular genre, say, women's fiction. If the non-compete clause is too broad, it could prevent the author from publishing more novels in that genre. Clearly that would be problematic.

Again, there are many terms in a book contract that I have not mentioned that are also of great consequence, but I wanted to point out these three, as they are often uniquely important to fiction writers and at times not fully understood.

When you're exploring different publishing options, consider what you value most: potential audience, ownership of the work, potential profit, creative control, prestige, legitimacy in academia, or legitimacy in the literary world. Be honest with yourself. While all of these issues may be important to you, prioritize. Make decisions that best align with your core concerns and goals. When you are making decisions about particular publishers, ask yourself these questions: Will they be good caretakers of my work? What is their track record? What are their marketing and sales plans? Do they share my vision? In short, do I trust them with my work? Fiction is highly personal. Authors are deeply invested in it, and more so than anyone else will ever be. Find the best home you can, and be careful about what agreements you sign.

Awards

If you're reading this book with an academic background, you probably know that there are many book and creativity awards given by different professional associations. These days, more and more authors are submitting social fiction for consideration. Don't be afraid to ask your colleagues or publishers to nominate your work or to self-nominate when that is allowed. I realize it can be difficult to think of our work in that light and awkward to ask others to get involved in the nomination process, but don't be shy. Writing the book was the most challenging part and you've shown that you're brave and vulnerable in releasing it. Now it's time to support your own work. In addition to academic awards, there are many different popular awards given for fiction each year, including general book awards with fiction categories, awards specifically for fiction, and awards for independently published books (defined in a myriad of different ways) or for specific genres (e.g., romance, historical fiction). Do an online search to see what your work may qualify for and toss your hat in the ring. A trade or academic publisher is usually willing to provide any book copies you may need for these purposes, although there may be entrance fees you need to cover. If you've used a hybrid publisher or have self-published, you should be able to buy copies of your book at cost (which is much lower than the list price).

Not only do awards make authors feel good, but they can help you market and sell your book. They can also attract agents and publishers. They create buzz. So go for it, and if you have an online platform or email list, share any victories with your followers. I do want to caution that even though I'm encouraging you to throw your hat in the ring, because you can't win unless you play, with equal force I want to remind you that winning awards isn't why we do this work, nor is it validation. We write because we have stories to tell. Furthermore, writing a work of fiction you're genuinely proud of is validation in itself. Whether or not any literary, traditional, or academic work wins awards depends on a highly subjective and political process. It is not "proof" that your work is or is not valid or good. So go for it, but don't become too invested in the outcome.

Evaluation Criteria

Something wonderful and terrifying happens when fiction is published: people respond to it. As I've noted throughout this book, readers may have any number of reactions to a work of fiction, including strong positive or negative emotional responses. In fact, the general readers most likely to comment on your work are those with extreme reactions—they love it or hate it. Why they love it or hate it can be a mystery, as we all have personal preferences in fiction and subjective experiences in storyworlds. Our work may resonate deeply with some readers who become engrossed in our stories and may completely fail to capture the interest of other readers. What it takes for readers to "like" it varies, but often includes whether they enjoyed the characters, if they thought the plot worked, the emotional response they had to the story, and their subjective evaluation of the writing quality. Works of fiction resonate with different readers, or don't, depending on all kinds of considerations. It's highly personal. For general readers, as fiction authors all we can do is work on our craft, seek feedback before publication, and put out work we feel strongly about. However, we are also researchers, and therefore we have to contend with academic evaluation too.

All research is evaluated, regardless of paradigm. In the case of social fiction, the process is more complex. It will be evaluated by general readers in the same way they evaluate other literary art, according to how much they "like" it. Paying attention to the features and strengths of literary writing reviewed in this book will help you create solid fiction that audiences are more apt to like; however, there are no guarantees given the subjectivity that goes into reading fiction. As a form of research, social fiction is also evaluated by the academic community. While there is no doubt that subjectivity plays a large role here too—from personal preferences to perspectives on what constitutes research—there are criteria we can use to help assess social fiction. It is increasingly important that we adapt these criteria as more graduate students and early career scholars take up this work. We need ways to assess this work that go beyond the personal preferences and research experiences of faculty at that person's institution. We need benchmarks that we can say an author hit or missed to varying degrees.

While it's tempting to evaluate social fiction based on qualitative research criteria, that's a mistake. As an art form, social fiction differs significantly from most qualitative research. Traditional qualitative research necessarily involves garnering data in some form and requires strict fidelity to that data. The data must be represented accurately. In social fiction, literary artifice and imagination are central to the process and may even constitute the entire generative act. Even when data are collected with a traditional method, artistic license is used to interpret and represent that data (see Table 9.1). In social fiction, the idea of accuracy is more complex. It is not about truth, but rather truthfulness—essence, resonance, authenticity, plausibility, and believability.

In previous works I've created evaluation criteria for arts-based research (ABR), including fiction, drawing on the work of many in the

TABLE 9.1. "Truth" in Traditional Qualitative Research versus Social Fiction

Traditional qualitative research	Accurate representation of data, fidelity to the data
Social fiction	Truthfulness—essence, resonance, authenticity, plausibility, believability

field. I've combined those criteria with the specific features of literary writing and developed this list of assessment criteria. However, please do not take these criteria as the "gold standard." The truth is that each social fiction project is different. Some criteria apply more and some apply less in evaluating any specific work. These criteria apply differently to projects based on the circumstances surrounding each work of fiction—what the author was trying to achieve and their approach. For example, "rich descriptions" may be pertinent in one novel, and part of how an author achieved verisimilitude, but they may be irrelevant in another novel that's more reliant on dialogue rather than on description. Moreover, there's always subjectivity involved in evaluating any piece of research, especially with fiction, which is a personal reading experience for each reader. There's no checklist we can simply tick off. For example, whether a reader becomes invested in a specific character is influenced by many things, including their personal preferences, their own life experiences, and so on. So while I offer some criteria that can be used to assess the quality of social fiction, in practice these will not apply to each project nor is my list complete. So even though as authors we can strive to achieve these benchmarks and as evaluators we can use them to assess others' work, we must take them with a grain of salt.

I've been offering lists of evaluation criteria for ABR in general and social fiction more specifically for more than a decade, and as I always say, it's a messy terrain in practice. I offer these criteria only to help professionals in academic settings who need to provide gatekeepers legitimate ways to evaluate their work (itself an act of legitimization). Really, the suggestions for how to assess social fiction, in terms of its strengths, historical and contemporary uses, and literary tools, have been reviewed throughout this book and are all ways that we can judge quality.

Verisimilitude

When readers enter into a work of fiction, they gain entry into a story-world or virtual reality. The story-world may be quite familiar to readers or someplace new. The creation of a virtual reality is a hallmark of quality in social fiction (Barone & Eisner, 1997, 2012). It is important that readers clearly see, feel, and imaginatively experience the virtual world. To accomplish this, authors incorporate empirical details that ring true for readers, building believable possible worlds. Capturing verisimilitude is what imbues a work of fiction with authenticity (de Freitas, 2004). Here are some questions to consider:

- Are there rich descriptions? Can you envision the people and places portrayed? Have details been incorporated into the descriptions? If so, do the details resonate as truthful?
- Does the dialogue ring true? Does it sound authentic? Can you clearly hear the characters' voices? Are they finely drawn?
- What is the mood of the story-world? Is it clear? How has it been created?

Sensitive Character Portrayals and Empathetic Engagement

Social research has a primary goal and the ethical responsibility to sensitively portray human experience (Cole & Knowles, 2001). This requires tapping into nuance and affording people their multidimensionality. Characters in fiction should be well developed. The thoughtful portrayal of characters fosters empathetic engagement in readers (Barone & Eisner, 1997, 2012; de Freitas, 2003). Therefore, the promotion of empathy is both a goal of social fiction and a standard by which to evaluate it.

Writers may portray characters in ways to suit these goals through the use of literary tools, as addressed in Chapter 3, and by making specific content choices aimed at promoting empathy. For example, fiction writers concerned with social justice issues can disrupt stereotypes and/or challenge dominant ideology through their creation of diverse characters and the experiences those characters have navigating certain issues or challenges. Questions to consider include:

- Are there rich character portrayals? Are the characters multidimensional? Do the characters seem authentic?
- Do you feel an emotional connection to the characters? Do you care about them? Do you feel sympathetic or empathetic toward them? Do you feel invested in what happens to them?
- Do primary characters have a full character arc? Is their story complete?
- Have the characters challenged any stereotypes or biases? How so?
- Have the characters helped you to learn something new about yourself or society? Have they exposed you to new ideas, experiences, or perspectives? Have they prompted personal reflection?

Structure and Narrative Coherence

We begin to build works of fiction by creating a structure. Through the structure, we relay the narrative. A structure is a way of organizing the story we wish to tell. Structure influences pacing. Compositional design elements should be chosen in accord with your specific goals (Barone & Eisner, 2012). Here are some questions to consider:

- Does the selection of the general structure (short story, novella, or novel) make sense? What kind of literary structure was used (e.g., three-part structure)? Does this way of organizing the story work well?
- How is the story paced?
- If a master plot has been used, is it recognizable? Has it been used in a unique way? Does it aid the emotional journey of the story? Has the master plot been subverted? If so, does that produce new insight?
- Does the plot make sense? Can you follow the plot?
- Does the story line make sense? Can you follow the story line scene by scene? Is it engaging?
- Are the scenes vivid? Did you feel like you were there, watching the action unfold? Is narrative writing used well to summarize and provide additional pertinent information? Does the balance

of scenic and narrative writing (or exclusive use of one) make sense? If there is a narrator, is that voice trustworthy?
- Does the ending provide closure and/or ambiguity? Are expectations met or challenged in ways that make sense? Were you satisfied? Does the ending leave you wanting more? Did you think about the story or characters after you finished reading?
- Is the entire work of fiction cohesive? Do all of the pieces of the narrative fit together? Is there a complete narrative arc?

Aesthetics, Artfulness, and Use of Literary Tools

A work of fiction is literary art. Therefore, it must work as a piece of art. As with other forms of ABR, it's important to consider the intrinsic beauty or artistic merit of the work (Bamford, 2005; Barone & Eisner, 2012; Butler-Kisber, 2010; Chilton & Leavy, 2014; Faulkner, 2009; Leavy, 2009, 2015, 2020b; Patton, 2002). The fiction has to be "good." Aesthetic power is created through the incisiveness, concision, and coherence of the final artistic output (Barone & Eisner, 2012; Chilton & Leavy, 2014, 2020). When a literary work has "deep aesthetic impact," then rigor has been achieved (de Freitas, 2004, p. 269). The audience must experience the artistic representation as truthful (Chilton & Leavy, 2014, 2020). An intertwining of authenticity and artfulness occurs in the audience experience. Some scholars suggest that the authentic *is* aesthetic (Hervey, 2004; Imus, 2001), as summed up in this quote: "the best art is the most honest, authentic art" (Franklin, 2011, p. 89). In those cases where you're drawing directly on data derived from traditional research practices, there may be a tension between creating good art and reporting research findings (Ackroyd & O'Toole, 2010; Saldaña, 2011). In these instances, you need to balance honesty with artistic license.

As reviewed in Chapter 3, there are many literary tools that can be used to strengthen writing, which all speak to stylist choices. For example, consider how themes and motifs are woven into the narrative, the establishment of tone, the use of language and sentence structure, the use of description, detail, and foreshadowing; and the use of metaphor, simile, symbolism, and juxtaposition. Some questions to consider:

- Did you enjoy the story?
- Are you engaged by it? Were you immersed in the story-world?
- Are themes and motifs well crafted?

- Are there rich, lustrous descriptions?
- What is the quality of the writing? Are literary tools used well? How about language, detail, foreshadowing, metaphor, simile, symbolism, and juxtaposition? Does the use of these tools enhance the story?
- Is it good art?

Personal Fingerprint or Creativity

Every writer has their own style. As with other forms of ABR, the personal fingerprint of the artist may thus be used to assess social fiction (Banks, 2008; Barone & Eisner, 1997, 2012). Artistic works have a *voice*. Writing fiction is about finding and expressing your voice. Cultivating a personal style takes time and skill that will be developed over a lifetime of practice. Your personal fingerprint and creativity are what makes your novel different from someone else's in the same genre and on the same topic. They still will not be alike, if each author has their own approach, their own trademark style. A writer's personal style develops from the suite of choices reviewed thus far—topic and content selection; thematic coverage; structure, including plotting and story lining; characterization; tone or mood; and the rigorous use of literary tools. Questions to consider:

- Is the work creatively rendered?
- Does the author have a specific approach to storytelling? Is there a distinct voice or style?
- What is their approach to using language?
- Does the story have personality? For example, does a sense of humor come through?
- Do you want to read another work of fiction by this author?

Substantive Contribution

As with any other research project, social fiction contains substantive content. As we learned earlier, a narrative is necessarily *about* something. Fiction can contribute to our understanding about a historical event or time, a culture or subculture, a certain kind of experience, and many other topics. Fiction can make various kinds of contributions to the particular subjects explored. These contributions may be in the form of generating new insights or learning, building micro–macro links, raising awareness, or cultivating compassion. Social fiction is intended to be useful. In this same vein, social fiction is well suited to public scholarship. People outside of the academy can read it. Some other questions to consider include:

- What have you learned from this work of fiction? Have you learned something new? Has something you previously thought been challenged?
- Are micro–macro links forged? Can you see the connections between the characters' lives and the larger context in which they live?
- Has the fictional work increased your awareness about a particular issue or about how different issues are connected to each other?
- Is the work of fiction about an important topic? Can reading this story benefit people?
- For what is this story useful?
- Could nonacademic stakeholders understand and engage with the work of fiction? Is it understandable? Is it available?

Ethical Practice

Ethical practice is an expectation in all research, regardless of paradigm, and can be used as a benchmark by which to assess social fiction or any form of ABR. The word "ethics" comes from the Greek word "ethos," which means *character*. Ethics refers to morality, integrity, fairness, and truthfulness (Leavy, 2017). There is an ethical substructure that impacts every aspect of the research process (Hesse-Biber & Leavy, 2011; Leavy, 2011, 2017) from topic selection through the representation and distribution of research findings. As an emerging and rapidly growing research practice, ethical issues are still being fleshed out. Some scholars have suggested that the very practice of any kind of ABR is in some respect both ethical and moral (Denzin, 2003; Finley, 2007).

First and foremost, if data are generated via traditional research practices with participants, all traditional ethical standards must be followed: institutional review board approval, first do no harm, informed consent, voluntary participation, and confidentiality, among others. With respect to confidentiality, you may consider creating composite characters to avoid revealing too much about any real person. Regardless of whether you've generated data with participants or writing is your entire act of inquiry, there are a couple of ethical issues all writers must pay attention to. First, it's vital to sensitively portray people and their circumstances. Aim for multidimensionality. Be sensitive and culturally competent when writing across differences. Challenge stereotypes. Second, is the issue of artistic license, mentioned earlier. When you are doing something to "make the art better" consider carefully the messages in the work. Always consider the kinds of representations you are putting into the world, which become a part of the collective imagination. A few questions to consider include:

- Is there an ethical or moral imperative in writing a narrative about the particular subject? Is it a timely topic? Is there a social justice imperative?
- If there are research participants, have standard ethical guidelines been followed?
- Are characters and their circumstances sensitively and compassionately portrayed? Are characters afforded multidimensionality? Is there sensitivity with respect to race, ethnicity, religion, gender, age, sexuality, and physical or mental health?
- What messages about different people or situations come through? What are the takeaway messages?

Conclusion

To me, there's nothing more immersive than entering into a new story-world, whether it's one I've created or one I get to visit through someone else's fiction. I love reading. I also love writing, especially fiction. It's an amazing feeling to create a new story-world that we can crawl into. When we do our job well, others can crawl into it too, and that's also an amazing feeling. Writing fiction brings boundless rewards. It's not always easy though. There's a lot of discipline involved in writing fiction. Doing the work is what opens us up to the possible moments of magic that are part of the creative process. Sharing our fiction isn't always easy either. It makes us vulnerable. To me, it's more than worth it.

For what it's worth, here's my advice. Be brave. Experiment. Get creative. Read. Read a lot. Write. Develop a writing discipline. Edit. Seek feedback. Learn to let go. And above all, develop your own relationship with your work that isn't dependent on anything external, positive or negative. That's how to keep the well of inspiration flowing freely.

I'll share one little secret with you too. Not only will readers have their own relationship with your work, but the relationship you have with it will change. Here's the thing, the words on the page won't change, but you will. You'll relate to your work from a year ago, 5 years ago, 10 years ago, and 20 years ago differently than you do now. I have some characters that were initially close to me in many ways. Now when I reread those works, I see them quite differently and I feel differently about them too. They haven't changed; I have. So do the best you can to write stories that ought to be written, to create characters that may hold your hand and the hands of others, let them go out into the world, and then, really let them go.

A final piece of advice. There's only one way to create fiction: write. Just write. As you do so, you will reinvent yourself, reimagine the world, and invite others to do the same.

> **SKILL-BUILDING EXERCISE** Assessing social fiction helps us to become better writers of social fiction. Read a work of social fiction (for example, you can read the full-length version of one of my works noted in this book or select something from the suggested readings in the Appendix). Using the evaluation criteria detailed in this chapter, write a one- to two-page assessment of the fictional work. What did the author do well? What could be improved?

> **RETHINK YOUR RESEARCH** Using the evaluation criteria reviewed in this chapter, assess the work of fiction you created based on your research. While it's difficult to honestly assess our own work, as researchers, we know assessment is an important part of the process. Go through the criteria one by one and evaluate how well you hit those benchmarks, bearing in mind which ones were most relevant to your project. Be both kind and ruthless. Use this process to help you revise or rethink your fictional work, whether you are continuing on with it or using it as a learning experience for the next project.

Appendix
Recommended Reading

In order to write fiction, one must read fiction. I suggest reading popular fiction in genres that interest you. That's something you can determine on your own. It's also important to read social fiction to get a sense of how other scholars do this work. If you're interested, you can read my fiction, which has been noted throughout this book. I've also compiled this brief list of social fiction on timely topics. Note that many of these books include more than one topic, so these are broad categorizations at best.

- **Education**
    - *Gen Ed* by D. G. Mulcahy
    - *Myron Oygold* by Jason Matthew Zallinger

- **Gender**
    - *Terra Ludus* by Toni Bruce
    - *Scars* by A. Breeze Harper
    - *Gender Optics* by Shalen Lowell

- **LGBTQIA**
    - *Jackytar* by Douglas Gosse
    - *Other People's Oysters* by Alexandra C. H. Nowakowski and J. E. Sumerau
    - *Cigarettes & Wine* by J. E. Sumerau
    - *Homecoming Queens* by J. E. Sumerau
    - *Palmetto Rose* by J. E. Sumerau
    - *Scarecrow* by J. E. Sumerau
    - *Via Chicago* by J. E. Sumerau

- **Race/Multiculturalism**
    - *Family History in Black and White* by Christine Sleeter
    - *White Bread: Anniversary Edition* by Christine Sleeter

- **Pandemics/Quarantine**
  - *Buried Together* by R. P. Clair
  - *October Birds* by Jessica Smartt Gullion

If you're interested in a literary arts-based practice that was not reviewed in this book, here are a few genre-specific books I suggest.
- *Autoethnography: Understanding Qualitative Research* by Tony E. Adams, Stacy Holman Jones, and Carolyn Ellis
- *Ethnotheatre: Research from Page to Stage* by Johnny Saldaña
- *Poetic Inquiry: Craft, Method and Practice* (2nd ed.) by Sandra L. Faulkner
- *Writing Ethnography* (2nd ed.) by Jessica Smartt Gullion
- *Writing for Performance* by Anne Harris and Stacy Holman Jones
- *Writing the Personal: Getting Your Stories onto the Page* by Sandra L. Faulkner and Sheila Squillante

References

Abbott, H. P. (2008). *The Cambridge introduction to narrative* (2nd ed.). Cambridge, UK: Cambridge University Press.

Ackroyd, J., & O'Toole, J. (2010). *Performing research: Tensions, triumphs and trade-offs of ethnodrama*. London: Institute of Education Press.

Adams, T., Holman Jones, S., & Ellis, C. (2015). *Autoethnography: Understanding qualitative research*. New York: Oxford University Press.

Bamford, A. (2005). The art of research: Digital thesis in the arts. Retrieved from *http://adt.caul.edu.au/etd2005/papers/123Bamford.pdf*.

Banks, S. P. (2008). Writing as theory: In defense of fiction. In J. G. Knowles & A. L. Cole (Eds.), *Handbook of the arts in qualitative research* (pp. 155–164). Thousand Oaks, CA: SAGE.

Banks, S. P., & Banks, A. (1998). The struggle over facts and fictions. In A. Banks & S. P. Banks (Eds.), *Fiction and social research: By fire or ice* (pp. 11–29). Walnut Creek, CA: AltaMira Press.

Barone, T. (2008). Creative nonfiction and social research. In J. G. Knowles & A. L. Cole (Eds.), *Handbook of the arts in qualitative research* (pp. 105–116). Thousand Oaks, CA: SAGE.

Barone, T., & Eisner, E. (1997). Arts-based educational research. In R. M. Jaeger (Ed.), *Complementary methods for research in education* (2nd ed., pp. 75–116). Chicago: American Educational Research Association.

Barone, T., & Eisner, E. W. (2012). *Arts-based research*. Thousand Oaks, CA: SAGE.

Behar, R. (1995). Introduction: Out of exile. In R. Behar & D. A. Gordon (Eds.), *Women writing culture* (pp. 1–29). Berkeley: University of California Press.

Berger, M. (1977). *Real and imagined worlds: The novel and social science*. Cambridge, MA: Harvard University Press.

Berns, G. S., Blaine, K., Prietula, M. J., & Pye, B. E. (2013). Short- and long-term effects of a novel on connectivity in the brain. *Brain Connectivity*, 3(6), 590–600.

Bochner, A. P., & Herrmann, A. (2020). Practicing narrative inquiry: II. Making meanings move. In P. Leavy (Ed.), *The Oxford handbook of qualitative research* (2nd ed., pp. 283–328). New York: Oxford University Press.

Bochner, A. P., & Riggs, N. (2014). Practicing narrative inquiry. In P. Leavy (Ed.), *The Oxford handbook of qualitative research* (pp. 195–222). New York: Oxford University Press.

Booth, W. (1961). *The rhetoric of fiction*. Chicago: University of Chicago Press.

Burawoy, M. (2004, August). *For public sociology*. Presidential Address at the American Sociological Association Conference, San Francisco, CA.
Burawoy, M. (2005). For public sociology. *American Sociological Review, 70*(1), 4–28.
Butler-Kisber, L. (2010). *Qualitative inquiry: Thematic, narrative and arts-informed perspectives*. Thousand Oaks, CA: SAGE.
Capote, T. (1966). *In cold blood*. New York: Signet Books.
Caulley, D. N. (2008). Making qualitative research reports less boring: The techniques of writing creative nonfiction. *Qualitative Inquiry, 4*(3), 424–449.
Cheney, T. A. R. (2001). *Writing creative nonfiction: Fiction techniques for crafting great nonfiction*. Berkeley, CA: Ten Speed Press.
Chilton, G., & Leavy, P. (2014). Arts-based research practice: Merging social research and the creative arts. In P. Leavy (Ed.), *The Oxford handbook of qualitative research* (pp. 403–422). New York: Oxford University Press.
Chilton, G., & Leavy, P. (2020). Arts-based research: Merging social research and the creative arts. In P. Leavy (Ed.), *The Oxford handbook of qualitative research* (2nd ed., pp. 601–632). New York: Oxford University Press.
Clandinin, D. J., & Rosiek, J. (2007). Mapping a landscape of narrative inquiry: Borderland spaces and tensions. In D. J. Clandinin (Ed.), *Handbook of narrative inquiry: Mapping a methodology* (pp. 35–75). Thousand Oaks, CA: SAGE.
Cleeton, C. (2021, May 7). On the power of fiction: 8 novels about little-known historical events. *Literary Hub*. Retrieved from *https://lithub.com/on-the-power-of-fiction-8-novels-about-little-known-historical-events*.
Clough, P. (2002). *Narratives and fictions in educational research*. Buckingham, UK: Open University Press.
Cohn, D. (2000). *The distinction of fiction*. Baltimore: Johns Hopkins University Press.
Cole, A. L., & Knowles, J. G. (2001). Qualities of inquiry: Process, form, and "goodness." In L. Nielsen, A. L. Cole, & J. G. Knowles (Eds.), *The art of writing inquiry* (pp. 211–229). Halifax, Nova Scotia: Backalong Books.
Collins, P. H. (2007). Going public: Doing the sociology that had no name. In D. Clawson, R. Zussman, J. Misra, N. Gerstel, R. Stokes, & D. L. Anderton (Eds.), *Public sociology: Fifteen eminent sociologists debate politics and the profession in the twenty-first century* (pp. 101–116). Berkeley: University of California Press.
Coser, L. A. (1963). *Sociology through literature: An introductory reader*. Englewood Cliffs, NJ: Prentice Hall.
Daiches, D. (1938). *Literature and society*. London: Victor Gollancz.
de Beauvoir, S. (1969). *The woman destroyed*. London: Collins.
de Freitas, E. (2003). Contested positions: How fiction informs empathetic research. *International Journal of Education and the Arts, 4*(7).
de Freitas, E. (2004). Reclaiming rigour as trust: The playful process of writing fiction. In A. L. Cole, L. Neilsen, J. G. Knowles, & T. C. Luciani (Eds.), *Provoked by art: Theorizing arts-informed research* (pp. 262–272). Halifax, Nova Scotia: Backalong Books.
de Freitas, E. (2007). Compos(t)ing presence in the poetry of Carl Leggo: Writing practices that disperse the presence of the author. *Language and Literacy, 9*(1).
De Jong, R. N. (1982). *A history of American neurology*. New York: Raven Press.
Denzin, N. K. (2003). Performing [auto]ethnography politically. *Review of Education, Pedagogy, and Curriculum Studies, 25*, 257–278.

Denzin, N. K., & Giardina, M. D. (2018). Introduction: Qualitative inquiry in the public sphere. In N. K. Denzin & M. D. Giardina (Eds.), *Qualitative inquiry in the public sphere* (pp. 1–14). New York: Routledge.
Denzin, N. K., & Lincoln, Y. (Eds.). (2000). *The SAGE handbook of qualitative research*. Thousand Oaks, CA: SAGE.
Dunlop, R. (2001). Excerpts from Boundary Bay: A novel as educational research. In L. Neilsen, A. L. Cole, & J. G. Knowles (Eds.), *The art of writing inquiry* (pp. 11–25). Halifax, Nova Scotia: Backalong Books.
Eisner, E. W. (1997). The promise and perils of alternative forms of data representation. *Educational Researcher, 26*(6), 4–10.
Ellis, C. (2004). *The ethnographic: I. The methodological novel about autoethnography*. New York: AltaMira Press.
Faulkner, S. (2009). *Poetry as method: Reporting research through verse*. Walnut Creek, CA: Left Coast Press.
Finley, S. (2007). Arts-based research. In J. G. Knowles & A. L. Cole (Eds.), *Handbook of the arts in qualitative research: Perspectives, methodologies, examples, and issues* (pp. 71–81). Thousand Oaks, CA: SAGE.
Fish, B. J. (2018). Drawing and painting research. In P. Leavy (Ed.), *Handbook of arts-based research* (pp. 336–354). New York: Guilford Press.
Franklin, R. (2011). *A thousand darknesses: Lies and truth in Holocaust fiction*. New York: Oxford University Press.
Freeman, M. (2007). Autobiographical understanding and narrative inquiry. In D. J. Clandinin (Ed.), *Handbook of narrative inquiry: Mapping a methodology* (pp. 120–145). Thousand Oaks, CA: SAGE.
Freytag, G. (1863). *Die technik des dramas*. Leipzig, Germany: Hirzel.
Geertz, C. (1973). *The interpretation of cultures*. New York: Basic Books.
Glenn, E. N. (2007). Whose public sociology?: The subaltern speaks, but who is listening? In D. Clawson et al. (Eds.), *Public sociology: Fifteen eminent sociologists debate politics and the profession in the twenty-first century* (pp. 213–230). Berkeley: University of California Press.
Goldman, A. H. (2013). *Philosophy and the novel*. New York: Oxford University Press.
Goleman, D. (1995). *Emotional intelligence: Why it can matter more than IQ*. New York: Bantam Books.
Goodall, H. L. (2000). *Writing the new ethnography*. Walnut Creek, CA: AltaMira Press.
Goodall, H. L. (2008). *Writing qualitative inquiry: Self, stories, and academic life*. Walnut Creek, CA: Left Coast Press.
Gullion, J. S. (2014). *October birds: A novel about pandemic influenza, infection control, and first responders*. Rotterdam, The Netherlands: Sense.
Gutkind, L. (1997). *The art of creative nonfiction: Writing and selling the literature of reality*. New York: Wiley.
Gutkind, L. (2012). *You can't make this stuff up: The complete guide to writing creative nonfiction—from memoir to literary journalism and everything in between*. Boston: Da Capo/Lifelong Books.
Harrison, F. V. (1995). Writing against the grain: Cultural politics of difference in the work of Alice Walker. In R. Behar & D. A. Gordon (Eds.), *Women writing culture* (pp. 233–245). Berkeley: University of California Press.

Harvey, M. R., Mishler, E. G., Koenan, K., & Harney, P. A. (2000). In the aftermath of sexual abuse: Making and remaking meaning in narratives of trauma and recovery. *Narrative Inquiry, 10*(2), 291–311.
Hervey, L. W. (2004). Artistic inquiry in dance/movement therapy. In R. F. Cruz & C. F. Berrol (Eds.), *Dance/movement therapists in action. A working guide to research options* (pp. 181–205). Springfield, IL: Charles C Thomas.
Hesse-Biber, S. N., & Leavy, P. (2005). *The practice of qualitative research*. Thousand Oaks, CA: SAGE.
Hesse-Biber, S. N., & Leavy, P. (2011). *The practice of qualitative research* (2nd ed.). Thousand Oaks, CA: SAGE.
Holman Jones, S., Adams, T. E., & Ellis, C. (Eds.). (2013). *Handbook of autoethnography*. Walnut Creek, CA: Left Coast Press.
Hussey, R. (2021). 20 great works of philosophical fiction. Retrieved from *www.bookriot.com/best-philosophical-fiction*.
Imus, S. (2001). Aesthetics and authentic: The art in dance/movement therapy. In *Proceedings of the 36th Annual Conference of the American Dance Therapy Association*. Columbia, NC: American Dance Therapy Association.
Iser, W. (1980). *The act of reading: A theory of aesthetic response*. Baltimore: Johns Hopkins University Press.
Iser, W. (1997). The significance of fictionalizing. *Anthropoetics III, 2*, 1–9. Retrieved from *www.anthropoetics.ucla.edu/ap0302/iser_fiction.htm*.
Janesick, V. J. (2001). Intuition and creativity: A pas de deux for qualitative researchers. *Qualitative Inquiry, 7*(5), 531–540.
John, E. (2016). Caring about characters. In G. L. Hagberg (Ed.), *Fictional characters, real problems: The search for ethical content in literature* (pp. 31–46). Oxford, UK: Oxford University Press.
Josselson, R. (2006). Narrative research and the challenge of accumulating knowledge. *Narrative Inquiry, 16*(1), 3–10.
Kim, J. (2006). For whom the school bell tolls: Conflicting voices inside an alternative high school. *International Journal of Education and the Arts, 7*(6), 1–19.
Kim, J. (2015). *Understanding narrative inquiry: The crafting and analysis of stories as research*. Thousand Oaks, CA: SAGE.
Kristof, N. (2014, February 15). Professors, we need you! *The New York Times*. Retrieved from *www.nytimes.com/2014/02/16/opinion/sunday/kristof-professors-we-need-you.html*.
Labov, W. (2006). Narrative pre-construction. *Narrative Inquiry, 16*(1), 37–45.
Lakoff, G., & Johnson, M. (1980). *Metaphors we live by*. Chicago: University of Chicago Press.
Leavy, P. (2009). *Method meets art: Arts-based research practice*. New York: Guilford Press.
Leavy, P. (2011). *Essentials of transdisciplinary research: Using problem-centered methodologies*. New York: Routledge.
Leavy, P. (2013). *Fiction as research practice: Short stories, novellas, and novels*. Walnut Creek, CA: Left Coast Press.
Leavy, P. (2015). *Method meets art: Arts-based research practice* (2nd ed.). New York: Guilford Press.
Leavy, P. (2016). *Blue*. Rotterdam, The Netherlands: Sense.

Leavy, P. (2017). *Research design: Quantitative, qualitative, mixed methods, arts-based, and community-based participatory research approaches*. New York: Guilford Press.

Leavy, P. (2019a). Introduction to the Oxford handbook of methods for public scholarship. In P. Leavy (Ed.), *The Oxford handbook of methods for public scholarship* (pp. 3–16). New York: Oxford University Press.

Leavy, P. (2019b). *Spark*. New York: Guilford Press.

Leavy, P. (2020a). *Film*. Leiden, The Netherlands: Brill.

Leavy, P. (2020b). *Method meets art: Arts-based research practice* (3rd ed.). New York: Guilford Press.

Leavy, P. (2021a). Introducing research methods and practices for popularizing research. In P. Leavy (Ed.), *Popularizing scholarly research: Research methods and practices*. New York: Oxford University Press.

Leavy, P. (2021b). Introducing methods for working with nonacademic stakeholders, teams, and communities. In P. Leavy (Ed.), *Popularizing scholarly research: Working with nonacademic stakeholders, teams, and communities*. New York: Oxford University Press.

Leavy, P. (2021c). Introduction to the academic landscape, representation, and professional identity. In P. Leavy (Ed.), *Popularizing scholarly research: The academic landscape, representation, and professional identity in the 21st century*. New York: Oxford University Press.

Leavy, P. (2021d). *Low-fat love: 10th anniversary edition*. Kennebunk, ME: Paper Stars Press.

Leavy, P. (2022). *Celestial bodies: The Tess Lee and Jack Miller novels*. Kennebunk, ME: Paper Stars Press.

Leavy, P. (in press). *The location shoot*. Berkeley, CA: She Writes Press.

Lesser, W. (2014). *Why I read: The serious pleasure of books*. New York: Farrar, Straus and Giroux.

Maines, D. (2001). Writing the self versus writing the other: Comparing autobiographical and life history data. *Symbolic Interaction*, 24(1), 105–111.

McNiff, S. (2018). Philosophical and practical foundations of artistic inquiry: Creating paradigms, methods, and presentations based in art. In P. Leavy (Ed.), *Handbook of arts-based research* (pp. 22–36). New York: Guilford Press.

Mills, C. W. (1959). *The sociological imagination*. New York: Oxford University Press.

Nell, V. (1988). *Lost in a book: The psychology of reading for pleasure*. New Haven, CT: Yale University Press.

Norris, J. (2009). *Playbuilding as qualitative research: A participatory arts-based approach*. Walnut Creek, CA: Left Coast Press.

Patton, M. (2002). *Qualitative research and evaluation methods* (3rd ed.). Thousand Oaks, CA: SAGE.

Paul, A. M. (2013, June 3). Reading literature makes us smarter and nicer: "Deep reading" is vigorous exercise from the brain and increases our real-life capacity for empathy. *Time*. Retrieved from http://ideas.time.com/2013/06/03/why-we-should-read-literature/print.

Prentice, D. A., Gerrig, R. J., & Bailis, D. S. (1997). What readers bring to the processing of fictional texts. *Psychonomic Bulletin and Review*, 4(3), 416–420.

Richardson, L. (2000). Writing: A method of inquiry. In N. K. Denzin & Y. S. Lincoln

(Eds.), *Handbook of qualitative research* (2nd ed., pp. 923–948). Thousand Oaks, CA: SAGE.

Robinson, J. (2005). *Deeper than fiction*. Oxford, UK: Clarendon Press.

Rodway, A. (1958). *The truths of fiction*. New York: Schocken Books.

Saldaña, J. (2003). Dramatizing data: A primer. *Qualitative Inquiry, 9*(2), 218–236.

Saldaña, J. (2011). *Ethnotheatre: Research from page to stage*. Walnut Creek, CA: Left Coast Press.

Saldaña, J. (2018). *Writing qualitatively: The selected works of Johnny Saldaña*. New York: Routledge.

Sarbin, T. R. (Ed.). (1986). *Narrative psychology: The storied nature of human conduct*. Westport, CT: Praeger.

Sinner, A., Leggo, C., Irwin, R., Gouzouasis, P., & Grauer, K. (2006). Arts-based education research dissertations: Reviewing the practices of new scholars. *Canadian Journal of Education, 29*(4), 1223–1270.

Spence, D. P. (1984). *Narrative truths and historical truths: Meaning and interpretation in psychoanalysis*. New York: Norton.

Stout, C. (2014, April). *Considering the bonds between narrative art and narrative inquiry*. Paper presented at the annual conference of the American Educational Research Association, Philadelphia, PA.

Tenni, C., Smyth, A., & Boucher, C. (2003). The researcher as autobiographer: Analyzing data written about oneself. *Qualitative Report, 8*(1), 1–12.

Thompson, H., & Vedantam, S. (2012). "A lively mind: Your brain on Jane Austen." *NPR Health Blog*. Retrieved from *www.npr.org/blogs/health/2012/10/09/162401053/a--lively-mind-your-brain-on-jane-austen.html*.

Todman, D. (2007). Letter to the editor: More on literature and the history of neuroscience: Using the writings of Silas Weir Mitchell (1829–1914) in teaching the history of neuroscience. *Journal of Undergraduate Neuroscience Education, 6*(1), L1.

Torres, J. T. (2021). Reliability in fiction. *Fiction Writers Review*. Retrieved from *https://fictionwritersreview.com/shoptalk/reliability-in-fiction*.

Turner, M. (1996). *The literary mind: The origins of thought and language*. New York: Oxford University Press.

Van Maanen, J. (2011). *Tales of the field: On writing ethnography* (2nd ed.). Chicago: University of Chicago Press.

Vickers, M. H. (2002). Researcher as storytellers: Writing on the edge—and without a safety net. *Qualitative Inquiry, 8*(5), 608–621.

Visweswaran, K. (1994). *Fictions of feminist ethnography*. Minneapolis: University of Minnesota Press.

Watson, A. (2016). Directions for public sociology: Novel writing as a creative approach. *Cultural Sociology, 10*(4), 1–17.

Watson, A. (2020). *Into the sea*. Leiden, The Netherlands: Brill.

Watson, A. (2021). Writing sociological fiction. *Qualitative Research*, pp. 1–16.

Wheeler, S. C., Green, M. C., & Brock, T. C. (1999). Fictional narratives change beliefs: Replications of Prentice, Gerrig, and Bailis (1997) with mixed corroboration. *Psychonomic Bulletin and Review, 6*(1), 136–141.

Wolcott, H. F. (2009). *Writing up qualitative research* (3rd ed.). Thousand Oaks, CA: SAGE.

Index

Note. *f, n,* or *t* following a page number indicates a figure, note, or table.

Academic publishers, 193–194, 197. *See also* Publishing process
Academic research and scholarship
  accessibility of, 8–9, 36–38
  challenges of doing fiction as, 38–39
  writing process and, 26–27
Aesthetics, 202–203
Afterwards, 65
Age of Discretion, The (de Beauvoir), 20
Agents, literary, 192–193, 197. *See also* Publishing process
All the Summer Girls (Donahue), 168
Alternative structures, 47, 167–179. *See also* Structure of social fiction
Anthropology, 21–22
Artfulness, 7, 16, 202–203
Arts-based research (ABR). *See also* Research process
  challenges of conducting, 39
  creative writing process and, 4–5
  ethical practice and, 204–205
  evaluation of social fiction and, 198–199, 199*t*
  overview, viii, 32–34
Assumptions, 15, 63
Audience
  evaluation criteria and, 197–205, 199*t*
  generating ideas, themes, and data for writing and, 44
  genre and, 52–53
  responses to creative writing by, 66–67
Autoethnography, 27, 30–32. *See also* Ethnography
Awards, 196–197
Awareness, 15

Back matter, 64–65
Backstory, 163–164. *See also* Flashbacks; Storytelling
Before-and-after story, 167. *See also* Alternative structures
Before–together–after story, 167–168. *See also* Alternative structures
Belief systems, 15–16, 44
Bias, 171, 189, 201. *See also* Stereotypes
BIPOC (Black, indigenous, and people of color), 21–22, 23
Blue (Leavy), 88–89
  excerpts from, 89–96
  reflection on, 96–97
Boy in the Striped Pajamas, The (Boyne), 25
Brain functions, 34–36, 41*n*
Bravery, 8, 206

Captured conversations, 58. *See also* Dialogue
Celestial Bodies (Leavy) collection, 56–57, 63–64, 111–112, 162–166. *See also* *Constellations* (Leavy); *North Star* (Leavy); *Shooting Stars* (Leavy); *Stardust* (Leavy); *Supernova* (Leavy); *Twinkle* (Leavy)
Central conflict, 68–69, 71–81, 84
Central metaphor. *See* Metaphors
Chapters, long, 123–149
Character arc
  evaluation criteria and, 201
  Low-Fat Love (Leavy) as an example to illustrate, 71–83, 84
  overview, 68–69

215

Characterization, 55–59. *See also* Characters; Style in writing
Characters
  Blue (Leavy) as an example to illustrate, 89–97
  data collection and generation for social fiction projects and, 44–45
  derivative rights to, 196
  empathetic understanding and, 12–13
  ethical practice and, 205
  evaluation criteria and, 200–201
  Film (Leavy) as an example to illustrate, 98–107
  gaps in fictional narratives and, 50
  historical fiction and, 23
  in a multiple viewpoint narrative, 168–169
  North Star (Leavy) as an example to illustrate, 162
  overview, 16, 55–59, 122, 206
  rising action and, 68–69
  self and social reflection and, 15
  series and, 165
  set-up and, 68
  Shooting Stars (Leavy) as an example to illustrate, 121–123, 163–164
  short stories and, 189
  Spark (Leavy) as an example to illustrate, 178
  tone and, 54
  Twinkle (Leavy) as an example to illustrate, 147–148
  types, 57
Citation system, 39
Climax, 46
Close reading, 34. *See also* Reading
Closure
  epilogues and, 64
  evaluation criteria and, 202
  series and, 166
  structure of social fiction and, 51–52
Coherence, 30, 201–202
Cohesion, 30, 202
Collaboration, 30, 182, 183
Collections. *See also* Series
  Low-Fat Love Stories (Leavy & Scotti) as an example to illustrate, 182–189, 184*f*
  short stories and, 181
Collins, Patricia Hill, 37
Combination in the fictionalizing process, 10–11
Compassion
  empathetic understanding and, 12–13
  historical fiction and, 25
  interiority and, 85
  in research practices, 12

Confidentiality, 205. *See also* Ethical considerations
Confrontation, 68–69, 110
Connected works of fiction. *See* Collections; Prequels; Sequels; Series
Consciousness raising, 44
Constellations (Leavy), 62, 112, 149–150, 164. *See also Celestial Bodies* (Leavy) collection
  epilogue from, 150–153
  reflection on, 154
Content, substantive, 203–204
Contests, 192, 196–197
Continuous unfolding action, 50
Copyediting
  Celestial Bodies (Leavy) collection as an example to illustrate, 165
  language and, 61
  publishing process and, 192–193
  self-publication and, 194
Copyright. *See also* Publishing process
  hybrid publishers and, 194
  overview, 195–196
  self-publication and, 194
Coser, Lewis A., 38
Cover design, 194
Creative nonfiction, 26–28
Creative writing process. *See also* Publishing process; Writing process
  building a structure and, 46–52, 49*t*
  characterization and, 55–59
  literary tools and, 59–64
  overview, 4–8, 16, 66–67, 163, 205–206
Critical consciousness raising, 44
Cross-pollination, 182
Cultural frames
  ethical practice and, 205
  narrative autoethnography and, 30–31
  narrative inquiry and, 30
Current events, 43

Data in social fiction. *See also* Field research; Generative act of writing; Interviewing; Literature review
  analysis of, 29–30
  collection and generation of, 44–45, 46*t*
  evaluation of social fiction and, 198–199, 199*t*
  generating ideas, themes, and data, 43–46, 45*f*, 46*t*
  Low-Fat Love Stories (Leavy & Scotti) as an example to illustrate, 183–184, 184*f*
de Beauvoir, Simone, 3, 20–21
Deep reading, 34. *See also* Reading

Der Spiegel magazine, 27
Derivative rights, 196
Description, 61–62, 200, 202–203
Detail, 61–62, 202–203
Dialogue. *See also* Interiority
  Blue (Leavy) as an example to illustrate, 89–97
  evaluation criteria and, 200
  Film (Leavy) as an example to illustrate, 98–107
  internal dialogue of characters, 13, 59
  language and, 60
  Low-Fat Love (Leavy) as an example to illustrate, 84
  Low-Fat Love Stories (Leavy & Scotti) as an example to illustrate, 189
  North Star (Leavy) as an example to illustrate, 161–162
  overview, 57–59
  reading aloud, 61
  Shooting Stars (Leavy) as an example to illustrate, 164
  Spark (Leavy) as an example to illustrate, 178
  Twinkle (Leavy) as an example to illustrate, 148
Diaries, 24
Discipline, 6–7, 8, 16, 182, 205–206
Document analysis, 44–45. *See also* Data in social fiction; Diaries; Literary arts practices
Dominant ideologies, 44
Dramatic arc, five-part, 46–47, 71–84. *See also* Structure of social fiction

Economic disadvantage, 23
Editing. *See also* Copyediting
  Celestial Bodies (Leavy) collection as an example to illustrate, 164–165
  language and, 60
  reader response and, 67
Embedded narrative, 169. *See also* Alternative structures
Emotional capital, 47
Emotional responses, 54–55, 201
Empathetic engagement
  evaluation criteria and, 200–201
  generating ideas, themes, and data for writing and, 44
  historical fiction and, 25
  interiority and, 59, 85
  literary neuroscience and, 35–36
  overview, 12–13, 16
  self and social reflection and, 15

Endings, 50–52, 202
Epilogues, 64, 149–154
Ethical considerations, 55, 200, 204–205
Ethnography. *See also* Autoethnography; Qualitative research
  creative nonfiction and, 27
  literary tools and, 59–60
  narrative inquiry and, 29–30
  overview, 28
  qualitative research and, 28
Evaluation of work, 197–205, 199*t*
Existentialism, 20–21
Expectations
  evaluation criteria and, 202
  genre, 52
  sequels and, 88
  series and, 166
  structure of social fiction and, 50–52
Exposition, 46

Falling action, 46
Feedback from others
  Celestial Bodies (Leavy) collection as an example to illustrate, 164–165
  evaluation criteria and, 197–205, 199*t*
  language and, 60–61
  Low-Fat Love Stories (Leavy & Scotti) as an example to illustrate, 182
  reader response and, 66–67
  writer's block concept and, 182
  writing groups and, 60–61
Feminist existentialism, 20–21
Fiction as a research practice. *See also* Social fiction
  challenges of conducting, 38–39
  fictionalizing processes, 10–11
  historical fiction, 22–25
  humanities and social sciences and, 19–22
  overview, 2, 3, 16, 18, 205–206
  publishing process and, 192–196
  qualitative research and, 28–32
  sociology and, 38
Field research, 32, 44–45. *See also* Data in social fiction; Research process
Fields of Play (Richardson), 27
Film (Leavy), 43, 88, 98–99
  excerpts from, 99–106
  reflection on, 106–107
First drafts, 60, 164–165
Fish, Barbara J., 4
Five-part dramatic arc, 46–47. *See also* Structure of social fiction
Flash fiction, 190*n*

218 • Index

Flashbacks
   Blue (Leavy) as an example to illustrate, 89–97
   Film (Leavy) as an example to illustrate, 98–107
   overview, 62–63, 162
Flexibility, 8
Foreshadowing
   Blue (Leavy) as an example to illustrate, 89–97
   evaluation criteria and, 202–203
   overview, 62–63, 122
   Shooting Stars (Leavy) as an example to illustrate, 122
   Supernova (Leavy) as an example to illustrate, 156
Forewords, 65
Formatting, 154
Fractured narratives, 169. *See also* Alternative structures
Frank, Anne, 24
Front matter, 64–65

Gaps in writing, 48, 50
Gender, 19–22, 23
General structure. *See* Novellas; Novels; Short stories; Structure of social fiction
Generative act of writing. *See also* Data in social fiction; Reflexive writing; Research process; Writing process
   evaluation of social fiction and, 198
   Low-Fat Love Stories (Leavy & Scotti) as an example to illustrate, 182–189, 184*f*
   overview, 45, 46*t*
Genre, 52–53, 196

Historical fiction, 22–25. *See also* Holocaust fiction
Holocaust fiction, 23–25. *See also* Historical fiction
Hours, The (Cunningham), 169
How to Eat a Cupcake (Donahue), 168
Human experience, 8, 9–12
Humanities, 19–22
Humor, 54, 156–162
Hurston, Zora Neale, 3, 21–22
Hybrid publishers, 194–195, 197. *See also* Publishing process

Ideas for writing, 43–46, 45*f*, 46*t*. *See also* Inspiration sources for writing
Identity, 21–22, 23

Imagination, reader, 13, 50
In Cold Blood (Capote), 27–28
Inciting incident
   Low-Fat Love (Leavy) as an example to illustrate, 71–81, 84
   overview, 84
   set-up and, 68
Inequality, 19–22, 23
Inquiry, 1–2, 4, 45, 46*t*. *See also* Narrative inquiry
Insider–outsider dichotomy, 32
Insight, 179, 201, 203–204
Inspiration sources for writing
   generating ideas, themes, and data, 43–46, 45*f*, 46*t*
   overview, 5–6, 16, 42–43, 162–163
   seeking, 7
   titles and, 65
   writer's block concept and, 182
Intent, 3–4
Interactions between characters, 57–59. *See also* Characters
Interiority
   Blue (Leavy) as an example to illustrate, 89–97
   empathetic understanding and, 13
   Film (Leavy) as an example to illustrate, 98–107
   Low-Fat Love (Leavy) as an example to illustrate, 81–83, 84–85
   Low-Fat Love Stories (Leavy & Scotti) as an example to illustrate, 189
   overview, 59, 85
Internal dialogue of characters. *See* Interiority
Interpretations
   empathetic understanding and, 13
   gaps in fictional narratives and, 50
   Low-Fat Love Stories (Leavy & Scotti) as an example to illustrate, 183–184, 184*f*
Interviewing. *See also* Data in social fiction
   data collection and generation for social fiction projects, 44–45
   Low-Fat Love Stories (Leavy & Scotti) as an example to illustrate, 182–183, 184*f*
   narrative autoethnography and, 32
Into the Sea (Watson), 14
ISBN, 194

Journal articles, 36–37, 39, 192. *See also* Academic research and scholarship
Journalism, 26–27
Journals, personal, 24
Juxtaposition, 64, 202–203

Kindle Direct Publishing (KDP), 194

Language
  description, detail, and specificity, 61–62
  dialogue and, 58
  evaluation criteria and, 202–203
  literary tools and, 59–61
  narrative inquiry and, 29
Learning
  arts-based research (ABR) and, 33
  evaluation criteria and, 201, 203–204
  generating ideas, themes, and data for writing and, 44
  literary neuroscience and, 34–36
  self and social reflection and, 14–15
LGBTQIA individuals, 23
Literary agents, 192–193, 197. *See also* Publishing process
Literary arts practices, 5–6. *See also* Arts-based research (ABR); Creative writing process; Social fiction
Literary Mind, The (Turner), 33
Literary neuroscience, 34–36, 41n
Literary structure. *See* Structure of social fiction
Literary tools, 59–64, 202–203. *See also* Description; Flashbacks; Foreshadowing; Language; Metaphors; Symbolism
Literature review, 44–45. *See also* Data in social fiction
Location Shoot, The (Leavy), 64, 168
Long chapters, 123–149
Looking for Alaska (Green), 167
Low-Fat Love (Leavy), 5, 14, 52, 65
  as an example of a traditional three-act structures, 69–86
  excerpts from, 71–83
  reflection on, 83–86
Low-Fat Love Stories (Leavy & Scotti), 182–184, 184f
  excerpts from, 185–188
  reflection on, 189

Magic
  Celestial Bodies (Leavy) collection as an example to illustrate, 163–166
  creative writing process and, 8, 16
Master plots. *See also* Plot
  character types and, 57
  evaluation criteria and, 201
  overview, 47

Meaning, 63
Meet cutes, 97
Metaphors
  Constellations (Leavy) as an example to illustrate, 154
  evaluation criteria and, 202–203
  overview, 63
  Supernova (Leavy) as an example to illustrate, 154–156
Micro–macro connections
  evaluation criteria and, 204
  generating ideas, themes, and data for writing and, 44
  interiority and, 59
  literary neuroscience and, 35
  metaphors and similes and, 63
  overview, 14
Mitchell, Silas Weir, 41n
Monologue, The (de Beauvoir), 20
Motifs, 53, 202–203. *See also* Themes
Mrs. Dalloway (Woolf), 169
Multidimensionality, 205
Multiple viewpoint narrative, 168–169. *See also* Alternative structures
Multiple-day narrative, 169–179. *See also* Alternative structures

Narrative, 8, 60, 68
Narrative arc, 165, 202
Narrative art, 29
Narrative autoethnography, 30–32. *See also* Autoethnography; Qualitative research
Narrative coherence. *See* Coherence
Narrative in social fiction, 48–50, 49t. *See also* Social fiction
Narrative inquiry, 29–30, 40n–41n. *See also* Inquiry; Qualitative research
Nausea (Sartre), 20
Nested story, 169. *See also* Alternative structures
Neuroscience, literary, 34–36, 41n
Newspaper reporting, 26–27
No Exit (Sartre), 20
Non-compete clause, 196
Nonfiction, creative, 26–28
North Star (Leavy), 112, 156–157, 164. *See also Celestial Bodies* (Leavy) collection
  excerpts from, 157–161
  reflection on, 161–162
Novel sequences, 109–110. *See also* Series
Novellas, 46, 181, 190n. *See also* Short stories; Structure of social fiction
Novels, 46, 190n. *See also* Structure of social fiction

220 • Index

October Birds (Gullion), 14
Online platforms for publishing, 192. See also Publishing process
Open form structures, 47, 110. See also Structure of social fiction
Oral histories, 27
Organization, 148–149

Pacing, 148–149, 201
Perseverance, 192
Personal interests, 43
Personal journals, 24
Perspective
  evaluation criteria and, 201
  historical fiction and, 25
  in a multiple viewpoint narrative, 168–169
  short stories and, 189
  social fiction and, 3–4
Phillips, Natalie, 34
Philosophy, 3, 19–21, 33–34
Plot. See also Structure of social fiction
  alternative structures and, 179
  character types and, 57
  evaluation criteria and, 201
  Low-Fat Love (Leavy) as an example to illustrate, 71–83
  master plots, 47
  North Star (Leavy) as an example to illustrate, 161–162
  overview, 47–48
  Spark (Leavy) as an example to illustrate, 179
  traditional three-act structures and, 68–69
Poetics (Aristotle), 46
Political consciousness raising, 44
Prefaces, 65
Preparedness, 192
Prequels, 87
Print-on-demand publications, 194, 195. See also Self-publishing
Prologues, 64
Protagonist. See Characters
Psychological processes, 85
Public scholarship, 8–9, 36–38
Publishing process
  awards and, 196–197
  evaluation criteria and, 197–205, 199t
  for fiction works, 192–196
  overview, 191
Purpose, 52–53. See also Themes

Qualitative research. See also Ethnography; Research process
  arts-based research (ABR) and, 32

evaluation of social fiction and, 198–199, 199t
Low-Fat Love Stories (Leavy & Scotti) as an example to illustrate, 182–189, 184f
metaphors and, 63
narrative inquiry and, 29–32
overview, 28–32
themes and motifs and, 53
verisimilitude and, 9, 28

Race, 21–22, 23
Reader response, 66–67, 197–205, 199f. See also Audience
Reading
  importance of, 205–206
  literary neuroscience and, 34–36
  process of reading and writing fiction and, 2
Realism
  dialogue and, 58
  evaluation criteria and, 200
  in fiction, 9–12
  qualitative research and, 28
  scenes and, 48–49
Reflection, 14–16, 35, 201
Reflexive writing, 28, 31–32, 45. See also Generative act of writing
Rejections in the publication process, 192–193
Relotius, Claas, 27
Re-plotting, 30
Representation
  ethical practice and, 205
  Low-Fat Love Stories (Leavy & Scotti) as an example to illustrate, 183–184, 184f
  writing as a generative act and, 45, 46t
Research process. See also Arts-based research (ABR); Generative act of writing
  arts-based research (ABR) and, 32–34
  creative writing as a part of, 4–8, 16, 26–28
  ethical practice and, 204–205
  evaluation and, 198
  publishing process and, 193–194
  qualitative research and, 28–32
  social fiction and, 8–9
  Spark (Leavy) as an example to illustrate, 169–179
  verisimilitude and, 9
  writing throughout, 1–2
Resolution
  Low-Fat Love (Leavy) as an example to illustrate, 81–83
  in open form structures, 110

overview, 69
structure of social fiction and, 46
Resonance
  character types and, 57
  in fiction, 9–12
  generating ideas, themes, and data for writing and, 44
Re-storying, 30
Revelation, 69, 81–83
Reviewers, 39, 197–205, 199*t*
Revisions, 60, 164–165
Richardson, Laurel, 27
Rising action
  Low-Fat Love (Leavy) as an example to illustrate, 71–81
  overview, 68–69
  structure of social fiction and, 46

Salzburg Global Seminar, 170
Sartre, Jean-Paul, 3, 19–20, 21
Scenes. *See also* Setting
  evaluation criteria and, 200, 201–202
  language and, 60
  long chapters and, 148–149
  North Star (Leavy) as an example to illustrate, 161–162
  open form structures and, 110
  overview, 48–50, 49*t*
  Shooting Stars (Leavy) as an example to illustrate, 163
  Twinkle (Leavy) as an example to illustrate, 148–149
Schindler's List (Keneally), 25
Scholarship. *See* Academic research and scholarship; Public scholarship
Science, 33
Scotti, Victoria, 183
Second Sex, The (de Beauvoir), 20
Self-reflection, 14–16, 35
Self-consciousness, 31–32
Self-disclosure in the fictionalizing process, 10–11
Self-publishing, 194. *See also* Publishing process
Sentence structure, 202–203
Sequels. *See also* Structure of social fiction
  derivative rights and, 196
  Film (Leavy) as an example of, 98–107
  overview, 47, 87–88
Series. *See also* Structure of social fiction
  Celestial Bodies (Leavy) collection as an example to illustrate, 111–112, 163–166
  Constellations (Leavy) as an example to illustrate, 149–154

derivative rights and, 196
North Star (Leavy) as an example to illustrate, 156–162
overview, 47, 109–110, 163–166
Shooting Stars (Leavy) as an example to illustrate, 112–123
Supernova (Leavy) as an example to illustrate, 154–156
Twinkle (Leavy) as an example to illustrate, 123–149
Setting. *See also* Scenes
  set-up and, 68
  Shooting Stars (Leavy) as an example to illustrate, 121
  Twinkle (Leavy) as an example to illustrate, 147–148
Set-up, 68, 110
Shooting Stars (Leavy), 49–50, 49*t*, 65, 112–113. *See also Celestial Bodies* (Leavy) collection
  excerpts from, 113–121
  reflection on, 121–123, 162–164
Short stories. *See also* Structure of social fiction
  Low-Fat Love Stories (Leavy & Scotti) as an example to illustrate, 182–189, 184*f*
  overview, 46, 181
  publishing process and, 192
  word counts and, 190*n*
Signposting, 148–149
Similes, 63, 202–203
Single-day narrative, 169. *See also* Alternative structures
Social fiction. *See also* Creative nonfiction; Creative writing process; Fiction as a research practice; Publishing process; Writing process
  challenges of doing fiction as research and, 38–39
  creative writing process and, 4–8
  empathetic understanding and, 12–13
  evaluation criteria and, 197–205, 199*t*
  historical fiction and, 22–25
  humanities and social sciences and, 19–22
  literary neuroscience and, 35
  micro–macro connections and, 14
  overview, viii–ix, 3–4, 16, 40, 205–206
  publishing, 192–196
  qualitative research and, 28–32
  self and social reflection and, 14–16
  strengths of, 8–16
  structure for, 46–52, 49*t*
  verisimilitude and, 9–12
Social justice research, 12, 43, 205

Social reflection, 14–16, 35
Social research, 28–32. *See also* Research process
Social sciences, 19–22
Sociology, 3–4, 14, 37–38
Sociology through Literature (Coser), 38
Sociopsychological processes, 59
Spark (Leavy), 169–171
 excerpts from, 171–178
 reflection on, 178–179
Specificity, 62
Stardust (Leavy), 112, 166. *See also Celestial Bodies* (Leavy) collection
Stereotypes
 characterization and, 55
 ethical practice and, 205
 evaluation criteria and, 201
 generating ideas, themes, and data for writing and, 44
 literary neuroscience and, 35
 self and social reflection and, 14–15
 social fiction and, 16
Stories, short. *See* Short stories
Story arc, 165, 202
Story line. *See also* Plot
 alternative structures and, 179
 evaluation criteria and, 201
 overview, 47–48
 Spark (Leavy) as an example to illustrate, 179
Story within a story, 169. *See also* Alternative structures
Storytelling
 arts-based research (ABR) and, 33
 creative nonfiction and, 26–27
 flashbacks and, 63
 Holocaust fiction and, 24–25
 human experience and, 8
 narrative inquiry and, 29
 North Star (Leavy) as an example to illustrate, 161–162
 overview, 162
 series and, 165
 Shooting Stars (Leavy) as an example to illustrate, 163–164
 Twinkle (Leavy) as an example to illustrate, 148
Structure of social fiction. *See also* Alternative structures; Novellas; Novels; Open form structures; Sequels; Series; Short stories; Traditional three-act structures
 endings, closure, and expectations, 51–52
 evaluation criteria and, 201–202
 master plots, 47

overview, 46–47
plot and story line, 47–48
scenes, narrative, and gaps, 48–50
style, 52–55
Style in writing. *See also* Voice in writing
 characterization and, 55–59
 evaluation criteria and, 203
 genre, 52–53
 overview, 52–55, 66, 163
 themes and motifs, 53
 tone and, 53–55
Submission for publication. *See also* Publishing process
 awards and, 196–197
 hybrid publishers and, 195
 overview, 192–194
Substantive content, 203–204
Sunrise over Hell (Ka-Tzetnik 135633), 25
Supernova (Leavy), 62, 63, 112, 154–155. *See also Celestial Bodies* (Leavy) collection
 excerpt from, 155–156
 reflection on, 156
Symbolism, 63–64, 189, 202–203
Sympathetic engagement
 evaluation criteria and, 201
 generating ideas, themes, and data for writing and, 44
 interiority and, 59, 85
 literary neuroscience and, 35–36
 overview, 12–13

Temporal gaps, 50. *See also* Gaps in writing
Testimonials, 24
Themes. *See also* Inspiration sources for writing
 evaluation criteria and, 202–203
 Film (Leavy) as an example to illustrate, 98–107
 generating ideas, themes, and data, 43–46, 45*f*, 46*t*
 genre and, 52–53
 Low-Fat Love Stories (Leavy & Scotti) as an example to illustrate, 189
 overview, 53
 series and, 112, 165
 Shooting Stars (Leavy) as an example to illustrate, 121, 164
 Supernova (Leavy) as an example to illustrate, 156
 Twinkle (Leavy) as an example to illustrate, 148
Thick description, 61. *See also* Description
Third-person narrative, 81–83, 84, 85

Thousand Darknesses, A (Franklin), 23
Three-act structures. *See* Traditional three-act structures
Titles, 65–66, 156
Tone in writing, 53–55, 156–162. *See also* Voice in writing
Topics, 43–46, 45*f*, 46*t*. *See also* Inspiration sources for writing
Trade publishers, 192–193, 197. *See also* Publishing process
Traditional three-act structures. *See also* Structure of social fiction
  Blue (Leavy) as an example of, 89–97
  Film (Leavy) as an example of, 98–107
  Low-Fat Love (Leavy) as an example of, 69–86
  overview, 47, 68–69
  plot and story line and, 48
Trilogies, 109–110. *See also* Series
Twinkle (Leavy), 112, 123. *See also Celestial Bodies* (Leavy) collection
  excerpts from, 123–147
  reflection on, 147–149, 164
Typesetters, 194

Values, 43
Van Maanen, John, 59–60
Vanity presses, 195
Verisimilitude
  evaluation criteria and, 200
  literary neuroscience and, 35
  overview, 9–12, 28
Via Chicago (Sumerau), 168–169
Visual analysis, 183–184, 184*f*

Visual arts, 7, 183–184, 184*f*
Voice in writing. *See also* Style in writing
  character types and, 57
  evaluation criteria and, 203
  overview, 53–55
  short stories and, 189
Vulnerability, 8, 31–32, 205–206

Woman Destroyed, The (de Beauvoir), 20–21
Word counts, 190*n*
Writer's block concept, 182. *See also* Discipline; Inspiration sources for writing
Writing as a generative act. *See* Generative act of writing
Writing conferences, 192
Writing groups, 60–61. *See also* Feedback from others
Writing process. *See also* Creative writing process; Publishing process; Social fiction
  building a structure and, 46–52, 49*t*
  characterization and, 55–59
  front and back matter, 64–65
  generating ideas, themes, and data, 43–46, 45*f*, 46*t*
  literary tools and, 59–64
  overview, 2, 42–43, 66–67, 163, 205–206
  style and, 52–55
  titles, 65–66

Yellow Wallpaper, The (Gilman), 41*n*

About the Author

Patricia Leavy, PhD, is an independent sociologist, novelist, and former Chair of Sociology and Criminology and Founding Director of Gender Studies at Stonehill College in Easton, Massachusetts. She is the author, coauthor, or editor of 40 nonfiction and fiction books, which have been translated into multiple languages. Her fiction has received many awards, including a recent first-place Firebird Book Award in Romance for *Celestial Bodies: The Tess Lee and Jack Miller Novels,* and an American Fiction Award for Inspirational Fiction, a Living Now Book Award for Adventure Fiction, and a National Indie Excellence Award for the novel *Spark*. Dr. Leavy has served as the creator and editor of 10 book series and is cofounder of the journal *Art/Research International.* For her work in the field of research methods, she has received honors including the Distinguished Service Outside the Profession Award from the National Art Education Association, the New England Sociologist of the Year Award from the New England Sociological Association, the Special Achievement Award from the American Creativity Association, the Significant Contribution to Educational Measurement and Research Methodology Award from Division D of the American Educational Research Association (AERA), the Outstanding Achievement in Arts and Learning Award from the Arts and Learning Special Interest Group of the AERA, and the Special Career Award from the International Congress of Qualitative Inquiry. The School of Fine and Performing Arts at the State University of New York at New Paltz has established the Patricia Leavy Award for Art and Social Justice in her honor. Dr. Leavy delivers invited lectures and keynote addresses at universities and conferences. Her website is *www.patricialeavy.com.*